Animal-Assisted Intervention

Angela K. Fournier

Animal-Assisted Intervention

Thinking Empirically

palgrave
macmillan

Angela K. Fournier
Psychology
Bemidji State University
Bemidji, MN, USA

ISBN 978-3-030-32974-7 ISBN 978-3-030-32972-3 (eBook)
https://doi.org/10.1007/978-3-030-32972-3

This Palgrave Pivot imprint is published by the registered company Springer Nature Switzerland AG.
The registered company address is: Gewerbestrasse 11, 6330 Cham, Switzerland

To family and friends, two-legged and four

Preface

This is a little book with some big ideas. The overall purpose is to promote empirical methods toward developing a deeper understanding of animal-assisted intervention—the practice of incorporating animals into procedures aimed at improving human health and well-being. Animals have been affecting our health and well-being throughout history. Inclusion in organized activities or treatments is a more recent development, with empirical investigations even more recent than that. Scholars have been thinking empirically about animal-assisted intervention for some time now, and the evidence base is growing. My aim in this book is to add fuel to the fire, introducing new ideas on measurement, experimentation, and interpretation. The premise is to move away from applied studies that focus solely on human outcomes and move toward more basic research, testing theory-driven hypotheses addressing the role of the animal in the intervention process. Content is centered around a deeper analysis of human–animal interaction and the animal as a key intervention component. To date, research focuses on the humans receiving the intervention and measures a wide array of human outcomes. There is very little study of just how humans and animals interact and which interactions with or features of the animal are therapeutic. In other words, we haven't examined whether the animal is a critical ingredient in animal-assisted interventions. My hope is that this book provides some ideas and methods for turning the microscope in that direction.

The book will be useful for scholars and practitioners in animal-assisted intervention. For academics, this book may validate the empirical work you are already doing and spur ideas for expansion. Perhaps you will think of new variables to investigate or new ways to investigate those you have already studied. Research on animal-assisted intervention is evolving, with studies gaining in rigor over time. Individual studies addressing a myriad of populations and outcomes are being summarized in systematic reviews and meta-analyses, providing a wider lens to see the big picture. Studies are shifting from largely applied, correlational studies that describe relationships to experimental studies testing hypotheses. In this book I propose another shift—from focusing exclusively on the intervention outcome to examining the intervention process. Several means for doing this are provided; hopefully it is just the beginning of a deep dive into the practice and purpose of human–animal interactions within animal-assisted intervention.

For practitioners of animal-assisted intervention—those of you who share your time, talent, and in many cases your four-legged family members—the hope is that this book inspires you to question the *how* and *why* of your work. In your own practice, you probably already see the effects of the work you and your animal(s) do. People doing animal-assisted therapy and learning likely gather pre–post data to determine client progress. Those doing animal-assisted activities probably note changes in recipients' affect, behavior, and attitude. My hope is that reading this book validates any current empirical inclination and pushes you further. Perhaps you will start thinking about just how it is that your animal assists you in helping others. Is it the way the animal looks or acts? Is it something about the species or breed? Are there certain clients who seem to benefit more from interacting with your animal than others? Are there certain behaviors your animal performs that foster health and wellness? Thinking empirically to ask these types of questions can inform your practice, allowing for even greater reach.

So here's to big ideas and moving our field forward. Working together to think empirically, we can demystify animal-assisted intervention and promote positive practices.

Bemidji, MN

Angela K. Fournier

Acknowledgments

Writing this book has been a wonderful experience and I'm grateful to everyone at Palgrave Macmillan for this opportunity for personal and professional growth. Thank you to Rachel Daniel, senior editor, for initiating the process, coordinating the proposal and review, and starting me on this adventure. Thank you to Madison Allums, editorial assistant, for working with me throughout the writing process, answering questions and providing guidance. And thank you to the production team for completing the process and turning my words into a beautiful book.

I've been fortunate to work on animal-assisted intervention through teaching, research, and clinical practice. I'm grateful to mentors, colleagues, and friends in each of these areas for their support and encouragement. Dr. E. Scott Geller was my doctoral mentor at Virginia Tech. As I'm writing this, he is starting his 50th year as a psychology professor. His dedication to teaching, learning, psychology, and science is awesome and I am grateful for his continued mentorship and support. I am thankful to Dr. Thomas Berry, who was my undergraduate mentor in psychology at Christopher Newport University and has remained a supportive mentor. Tom has been instrumental in developing the ideas and conducting much of the research discussed in the book. I'm grateful for his support and collaboration. After taking a hiatus from studying human–animal interaction, a bright graduate student renewed my interest with her master's thesis on equine-assisted therapy. That student, Elizabeth Letson, has since become my colleague in delivering and researching animal-assisted interventions. As owner of Eagle Vista Ranch & Wellness Center (EVR), Liz has partnered with me to conduct both basic and applied research. She courageously turns her pasture into a laboratory and works with my students and me to study human–horse interactions. I'm grateful for her passion and curiosity around helping people through animals and nature, and her kind, patient collaboration on research. Thank you to Jennifer Laitala, equine specialist at EVR. Jen has given her time and energy to research projects, meetings with students, and brainstorming sessions. I appreciate her perspective and am grateful for her collaboration.

The empirical studies described in this book were possible because of the many people who volunteered to participate in research. To the inmates in the PenPals program, Pet Partners practitioners, Great River Rescue staff and volunteers, animal-assisted intervention clients, and university students who volunteered your time and reported on your experiences—thank you. You have made an important contribution to the science and practice of animal-assisted intervention. Many students have worked with me over the years, studying human–animal interaction. I'm grateful for their curiosity in developing ideas and their assistance in data collection, analysis, and interpretation. I am particularly grateful to Emma Pasiuk and Lori Winston, who went above and beyond any course requirements to help with research. They have exceeded my expectations and I can't wait to see how they contribute to the field. I'm grateful to faculty and administration at Bemidji State University for supporting my research. I am particularly thankful to my colleagues in the psychology department. They have encouraged me to conduct this research, promoted studies in their courses, sent me students interested in serving as research assistants, and agreed to having all kinds of animals in our shared laboratory space. I'm grateful for their friendship and support.

I've also been blessed with wonderful support from my family. My parents always encouraged my curiosity and raised me to love both animals and science. I'm grateful for their love and support. My daughter Mia inspires me every day to make a difference in the world. She is patient while I write and has been known to pick up a clipboard occasionally to try out an observation technique. I'm thankful for her support and understanding when I needed time to write. My husband Justin is a more supportive partner than I could imagine. He listens to my ideas, provides supportive feedback, and is happy to take over family responsibilities to support my work. I'm thankful every day that he is by my side. And last but certainly not least, I am grateful for the animals. Animals in my personal life have inspired me to pursue this line of inquiry and animals in research studies have contributed greatly to developing the ideas in this book.

A great deal of the research discussed in the book, and all of the writing, took place in Bemidji, MN, USA. This area is located on traditional, ancestral, and contemporary lands of Indigenous people. The Bemidji area is the original homeland of the Ojibwe and Dakota. It is important to acknowledge the painful history of genocide, forced assimilation, and efforts to alienate the Indigenous inhabitants from their territory, and I honor and respect the many diverse Indigenous peoples still connected to this land. I am humbled to live and work in this special place and grateful for Indigenous community members and colleagues who broaden my perspective every day.

Contents

About the Author

Angela K. Fournier holds a PhD in clinical psychology from Virginia Tech. She is a licensed psychologist in Minnesota and professor in the department of psychology at Bemidji State University. She is certified in equine-assisted psychotherapy and learning (EAP) and co-facilitates EAP at Eagle Vista Ranch & Wellness Center in Bemidji, MN. As director of the Human–Animal Interaction Laboratory, she conducts studies into the psychological processes and outcomes of human–animal interaction, focusing on development of theory and validated measures.

Abbreviations

AAA	Animal-Assisted Activity
AAI	Animal-Assisted Intervention(s)
AAL	Animal-Assisted Learning
AAT	Animal-Assisted Therapy
ANOVA	Analysis of Variance
APA	American Psychological Association
BSU	Bemidji State University
CBT	Cognitive-Behavioral Therapy
EAGALA	Equine-Assisted Growth and Learning Association
EAP	Equine-Assisted Psychotherapy
EVR	Eagle Vista Ranch & Wellness Center
HAI	Human–Animal Interaction
HAIS	Human–Animal Interaction Scale
HHIS	Human–Human Interaction Scale
ISAZ	International Society for Anthrozoology
MDMS	Multidimensional Mood Scale
SUDS	Subjective Units of Distress Scale

List of Figures

List of Tables

CHAPTER 1

Introduction

Abstract This chapter introduces the concept of animal-assisted intervention (AAI), which includes animal-assisted therapy (AAT; e.g., psychotherapy, occupational therapy), animal-assisted education and learning, and animal-assisted activities (AAAs). A brief review of the literature conveys that AAI is prevalent and has a significant impact on society, but there are important gaps in our understanding. Despite an increasing number of studies showing positive outcomes, literature in this area consistently calls for (1) rigorous experimental research to test hypotheses, and (2) an explanatory theory or framework from which to study AAI. This chapter will provide justification for new approaches, including the need for reliable and valid instrumentation, experimental laboratory research, and a conceptualization of the role of the animal in the intervention process. The underlying theme in addressing these limitations is to bring a closer examination of human–animal interaction (HAI) into research on AAI.

Keywords Animal-assisted intervention • Human–animal interaction

My work in animal-assisted intervention (AAI) began in graduate school. I was studying clinical psychology at Virginia Tech and a nearby prison had implemented a prison-dog program (FETCH a Cure 2018). Puppies that would eventually become service dogs were living with inmates for their first year of life. The inmates raised them and began their behavioral

A. K. Fournier, *Animal-Assisted Intervention*,
https://doi.org/10.1007/978-3-030-32972-3_1

training. The program was deemed successful; puppies were healthy and well prepared for service training after their time in prison. People were certain the program was having positive effects on the inmates and wanted evidence. I was fortunate enough to serve as a research assistant, surveying and interviewing inmates in the program. With my first visit to the prison, I was hooked. It was amazing to see men who had been incarcerated and deemed unsafe for society, isolated and hardened by the experience, light up when talking about the dogs in their care. This was true of the prison staff as well; everyone loved the dogs and reported the program was having a positive impact on the inmates. We studied the program, trying to capture this impact.

At the time, prison-based animal programs were popping up in prisons across the U.S. But implementation preceded any scholarship addressing which variables are impacted, for the inmates, the facility, or the animals. This is a theme in AAI work in general; programs are implemented first and then we get curious about the impact they're having and try to guess what that impact might be. Unsure of just what this program was doing for the inmates, we cast a wide net. We gathered data on psychosocial factors like self-esteem and optimism and assessed symptoms for all kinds of psychological disorders (e.g., depression, anxiety, post-traumatic stress disorder). Naturally, we predicted each of these would be improved as a function of the program. To our surprise, these variables did not change much from before working in the program (i.e., pretest) to after (i.e., posttest). It turns out the inmates selected for the program were some of the healthiest, most well-adjusted inmates in the facility. They already had high self-esteem, were relatively optimistic, and didn't have much in the way of psychological symptoms to begin with.

From this experience, I knew that I wanted to continue research in this area and that it would be an exciting challenge to determine just how animals impact our physical and mental health. This led to my dissertation research which involved investigating another prison-dog program at a different prison. Dogs from an animal shelter were living in the prison for several weeks while the inmates trained them in basic obedience. The dogs left prison with better behavior and were adopted by families in the community. The question was: did the program impact the inmates? Taking a lesson from the previous study, I chose not to measure psychopathology. Inmates selected for the program were likely the best of the best and probably would not endorse symptoms of mental illness. Instead, I measured social functioning and progress in the prison's therapeutic community. I found improvements in both, from pretest to posttest, in comparison to a wait-list control group. I couldn't wait to share my findings with my dissertation committee; I had studied this amazing program and found significant results. During my oral defense they acknowledged the significant findings and then promptly raised the question that would eventually become my research program—*how*? *How* did working in the program—this AAI—impact social functioning? *Why* did social sensitivity increase for the inmates in the program while it decreased for inmates on the wait list? This book is written with these questions in mind: what effect do animals have on human health and well-being, and how or why do these effects occur?

Definitions

Animal-assisted interventions (AAIs) are events, programs, or processes in which people engage with animals for some physical, social, emotional, or cognitive outcome (Animal-Assisted Intervention International 2016). AAI is a broad field that includes AAAs aimed at providing comfort and improving quality of life; animal-assisted education or learning wherein animals are involved in a process to obtain academic or educational goals; or animal-assisted therapy (AAT) in which animals are part of a treatment process (American Veterinary Medical Association 2019). Each of these activities involve engaging animals in a process for the promotion of human health and/or well-being. Throughout the book, I refer to AAI in general; the goal is to spur empirical thinking about interventions that include animals, whether the intervention is an activity or a treatment of some kind.

In the most basic sense, AAI includes human–animal interaction (HAI), which can be defined broadly as any interaction between a human and a nonhuman animal. Anthrozoology is the scholarly study of HAI, including scholars from disciplines within the natural sciences (e.g., biology, environmental studies), social sciences (e.g., psychology, social work), and humanities (e.g., philosophy, history, literature). Anthrozoologists attend to a broad array of interactions between humans and animals, including those that are beneficial to the human and/or animal (e.g., pet ownership, AAI), harmful interactions (e.g., animal cruelty and abuse, animal attacks on humans), forms of entertainment (e.g., zoos, circuses, animal racing or fighting), and interactions where the animal appears to be absent (e.g., wearing fur or leather, eating meat).[1] As a clinical psychologist I study HAI as they relate to human health and well-being. Specifically, I study the processes and outcomes of AAI, a practice dating back to at least the 1700s.

History of Practice and Research

While humans surely engaged with animals for some benefit going back thousands of years, employing animals in health as we know it today dates back to the late 1700s. At that time, psychiatric patients were noted to benefit from caring for animals such as rabbits and poultry at the York Retreat in England (Tuke 1813). In 1860, Florence Nightingale, the founder of modern nursing, wrote about animals aiding in the relaxation of children and adults in psychiatric hospitals (Nightingale 1860). Regarding mental health, there are reports of using dogs in psychotherapy dating back to Sigmund Freud. Patients reported he frequently offered comments and interpretations through his dog Jofi (e.g., Grinker 1979). Boris Levinson is credited with carrying out the first formal use of animals in therapy (Levinson 1969), after discovering the effects of his dog Jingles on his patients (Levinson 1962).

Formal AAI research is relatively young, dating back to the mid-twentieth century. Hooker et al. (2002) review the history of using animals in health settings. Levinson presented his findings from using Jingles in child psychiatry at the 1961 American Psychological Association convention. Having recognized companion animals as influential in human psychological functioning, he called for research on the benefits of pets (Levinson 1978). Two psychiatrists at Ohio State University—Sam and Elizabeth Corson—were the first to collect quantitative data, conducting pilot studies with animals in hospital settings (Corson et al. 1975). The research expanded to nursing home settings, revealing physical, psychological, and social outcomes (Corson and Corson 1978). From there, research expanded to investigations of pet ownership and physical health.

Perhaps most well known is a study by Friedmann et al. (1980) on the survival rate of patients after myocardial infarction. Results showed patients with pets had a much greater survival rate. Research on AAI expanded in the 1990s, with nursing studies finding associations between the presence of dogs and lowered blood pressure (Harris et al. 1993). Potential mechanisms for the effect included distraction, social stimulation, and

[1] The latter is referred to as the *absent referent* (Adams 2015).

increased enjoyment. For greater detail, see writings on the history of the human–animal bond (Hines 2003; Serpell 2011), HAI research (Beck et al. 2018), and AAI research (Altschiller 2011; Hooker et al. 2002; McCardle et al. 2011).

Scientist-Practitioner Approach

Animals are incorporated into interventions in a wide array of helping professions. The *therapy* in AAT can include but is not limited to psychotherapy or counseling, social work, physical therapy, recreational therapy, occupational therapy, or speech therapy. Each of these is a practical treatment driven by science. The principles and practices are based on evidence gathered from scientists conducting empirical research; the treatment is delivered by trained practitioners. This illustrates two, often separate, roles in intervention work—researchers and practitioners. Graduate programs can produce professionals in one role or another. However, programs can also be designed to produce scientist-practitioners—professionals skilled in both areas.

As a scientist-practitioner in clinical psychology, I am trained to provide *clinical services* in psychology (i.e., assessment, diagnosis, and treatment of psychological disorders) and conduct *empirical research* in my field (e.g., conduct studies investigating the efficacy of psychological treatments). Referred to as the Boulder model (American Psychological Association 1949), this approach promotes both research and practice in psychology. Not without its critics (e.g., Frank 1984), the Boulder model can inform our work in AAA, AAT, and animal-assisted learning (AAL).

Perhaps because AAIs are modalities within a professional practice (e.g., equine-assisted psychotherapy is a modality for delivering psychotherapy), AAI *practice* has preceded and dominated AAI *research*. The number of certification/training programs and trained professionals in the clinical practice of AAI is much greater than programs and professionals in the scientific inquiry of AAI. This is certainly related to a lack of training programs in field-specific AAI. Programs tend to train practitioners to use animals in interventions in general (e.g., certification programs to incorporate dogs in healthcare settings) rather than within a specific field. For example, someone who wants to use dogs in the delivery of occupational therapy would first undergo graduate training in occupational therapy and then receive additional training in canine-assisted intervention. But at the time of this writing, there are no graduate programs in canine-assisted occupational therapy. This is similar to my education and training experience—I earned a PhD in clinical psychology and then became certified in equine-assisted psychotherapy. In this way, practitioners receive training in two separate areas, and may be required to integrate the two for clinical practice on their own. Many training programs in medicine and allied-health focus on practical delivery of health services rather than scientific understanding and inquiry. This is also true of training and certification programs for AAI; those enrolled receive education and training in practical skills rather than gathering data and testing hypotheses.

A scientist-practitioner approach would emphasize the importance of both practical skills and original research. I am not suggesting that everyone in AAI should be both a practitioner and a researcher. Rather, the field as a whole must evolve as science-driven. Similar to the Boulder model in psychology, we can build the field from a scientific foundation. The field must include practitioners and researchers and would benefit from professionals who can do both.

My identity as a scientist-practitioner elicits a curiosity about AAI that has informed my own teaching, research, and clinical work. Practicing equine-assisted psychotherapy allows me to see the AAI process up close. It brings up many questions that my students and I can test in the laboratory. Findings from laboratory studies then inform subsequent therapy practices. Because I am trained in both roles—practitioner and researcher—I often move back and forth between two ways of thinking. I believe in the power of engaging with animals for health and well-being and I'm curious about just how and why animals help us. As I see it now, we have a plethora of practitioners who believe in the process and provide animal-assisted services. We also have a strong group of scientists engaged in empirical work to understand the process and inform effective practice. This book is written for both audiences, aimed at providing empirical examples and spurring new ways of thinking about AAI process and outcome.

Thinking Empirically About Intervention Components

Despite studies showing positive outcomes from interventions with animals, scholars suggest much of the research lacks rigor necessary to conclude that AAI results in reliable outcomes (Griffin et al. 2011). Investigations are largely conducted in applied settings, with correlational or quasi-experimental methods (e.g., Calvo et al. 2016; Klontz et al. 2007). While studies of this nature are useful in describing relationships between variables, internal validity necessary to make cause-and-effect claims is limited (Anestis et al. 2014). For example, one-group pretest–posttest studies are fairly common, wherein patients receive AAI while reporting symptoms before and after. If reported symptoms are improved from pretest to posttest, we might conclude the intervention worked to improve symptoms. However, there are other potential explanations for the change in symptoms. Participants could have experienced some other event between pretest and posttest (i.e., history), they may have changed in some way (i.e., maturation), or they could have gotten better on their own (i.e., spontaneous recovery) (Cook and Campbell 1979). Each of these must be ruled out before making conclusions about the AAI's efficacy.

AAI is a complex process with many variables. The intervention includes three or more living organisms—patient, intervention facilitator (e.g., animal handler, social worker), and therapy animal(s). Each of these organisms brings its own personal factors, such as temperament and learning history, that impact process and outcome. Each intervention also occurs in a specific time and place; situational factors can interact with personal factors. We can think of an AAI session as a complex system; understanding which factors may have caused an outcome is a complex undertaking. Research is needed to examine each of these variables in order to determine specific effects.

To move toward a better understanding, basic research in AAI is necessary, identifying and parceling out individual factors to test their effects. My students, colleagues, and I have focused on one particular facet of AAI—the behavioral interactions that occur between humans and animals during intervention. We study the specific actions that occur during AAI. Through description and analysis, we're learning more about which kinds of interactions may be more or less beneficial. Our research is described throughout the book to provide examples of thinking empirically about this complex process.

Research Reported Here

This book is organized into chapters based on empirical concepts and potential areas of inquiry. Content includes review of previous research, discussion of strengths and weaknesses in our current understanding of AAI, and suggestions for thinking empirically about AAI. Throughout the book, I illustrate points by describing research conducted by my team and I at the Human–Animal Interaction Laboratory (HAIL). I describe several studies conducted in the university laboratory and in off-campus applied settings. The laboratory is a collaboration between my students and I in the department of psychology at Bemidji State University, Dr. Thomas Berry and students in the department of psychology at Christopher Newport University, and Liz Letson and Jen Laitala at Eagle Vista Ranch & Wellness Center (EVR). EVR is a private-practice counseling center providing AAT, specializing in equine-assisted psychotherapy and learning (EAP). Liz Letson, a licensed professional clinical counselor, is the owner and founder; Jen Laitala is the lead equine specialist. Liz and Jen have partnered with me to conduct both basic and applied research investigating AAI. I'll describe correlational studies in which we have tested relationships between variables within a de-identified archival client database, as well as experimental work in which the horse arena served as a laboratory to test hypotheses with college-student volunteers.[2]

These studies are included to demonstrate how a question could be addressed empirically. Because the sample sizes are relatively small and homogeneous, they are not intended to and should not be interpreted as *the truth about* or *the way to do* empirical AAI work. Instead, they are meant to provide an example and inspire ideas for future research.

Human–Animal Dichotomy

Throughout the book, I suggest the importance of and provide examples of methods to study HAI as a construct within AAI. I recognize the term HAI is redundant, in the sense that humans *are* animals. The terms *nonhuman animals*, *other animals*, *other-than-human animals*, and *animals that are not human* are sometimes used to distinguish between people and pets, but these terms can also be problematic. Each of these terms makes humans the default and groups everything that is not human together, a form of othering that maintains systems of oppression. This is especially important in issues of animal welfare and animal rights. While this book does not address either of these important topics, it is critical to remember the issues addressed in this book involve interactions between beings of the same kingdom—the animal kingdom. I use the term human–animal interaction as, at the time of this writing, it is the term often used when discussing AAI and related topics.

[2] All research reported was reviewed and approved by an institutional review board, ensuring ethical treatment of human subjects in research. Research where animals were manipulated was reviewed and approved by an institutional animal care and use committee, which ensures ethical treatment of animals in research.

Organization of the Book

The book is organized into chapters based on empirical concepts or methods. Chapter 2 introduces the concept of measurement and the need for valid and reliable measurement instruments. I introduce the Human–Animal Interaction Scale (HAIS), an instrument we use in the HAI laboratory to describe and analyze behavioral interactions that occur during intervention. In Chap. 3, I discuss the concept of intervention dose, review the literature on AAI dose to date, and introduce alternative ways of operationalizing the construct. The chapter includes an introduction to dose–response relationships, addressing the relationship between differing quantities of HAI and intervention outcome. Chapters 4 and 5 examine the specific role of the animal in AAI, suggesting animals can elicit an anodyne effect or serve as an intervention agent. Previous research is reviewed suggesting these roles are present in AAI; empirical research is described in which these specific roles have been targeted. In Chap. 6, I discuss the citizen-science approach, suggesting we explore it as a method for large-scale data collection on HAI and AAI. Chapter 7 provides a summary, conclusions, and recommendations for thinking empirically about AAI research and practice.

References

Adams, C. J. (2015). *The sexual politics of meat: A feminist-vegetarian critical theory* (25th Anniversary edition). New York, NY: Bloomsbury.

Altschiller, D. (2011). *Animal-assisted therapy.* Santa Barbara, CA: Greenwood Publishing.

American Psychological Association. (1949). *Training in clinical psychology.* Conference on graduate education in clinical psychology, Boulder, CO.

American Veterinary Medical Association. (2019). Human-animal bond. Retrieved from https://www.avma.org/kb/resources/reference/human-animal-bond/pages/human-animal-bond-avma.aspx.

Anestis, M. D., Anestis, J. C., Zawilinski, L. L., Hopkins, T. A., & Lilienfeld, S. O. (2014). Equine-related treatments for mental disorders lack empirical support: A systematic review of empirical investigations. *Journal of Clinical Psychology, 70*(12), 1115–1132.

Animal-Assisted Intervention International. (2016). Animal-assisted intervention. Retrieved from http://www.aai-int.org/aai/animal-assisted-intervention.

Beck, A. M., Barker, S., Gee, N. R., Griffin, J. A., & Johnson, R. (2018). The background in human-animal interaction (HAI) research. *Human-Animal Interaction Bulletin, 6.*, Special Edition, 47–62.

Calvo, P., Fortuny, J. R., Guzmán, S., Macías, C., Bowen, J., García, M. L., et al. (2016). Animal assisted therapy (AAT) program as a useful adjunct to conventional psychosocial rehabilitation for patients with schizophrenia: results of a small-scale randomized controlled trial. *Frontiers in psychology, 7*, 631.

Cook, T. D., & Campbell, D. T. (1979). *Quasi-experimentation: Design and analysis issues for field settings*. Boston, MA: Houghton Mifflin Company.

Corson, S. A., & Corson, E. (1978). Pets as mediators of therapy. *Current Psychiatric Therapy, 18*, 195–205.

Corson, S. A., Corson, E. O., Gwynne, P. H., & Arnold, L. E. (1975). Pet facilitated psychotherapy in a hospital setting. *Current Psychiatric Therapy, 15*(8), 277–286.

FETCH a Cure. (2018). *Pen Pals*. Retrieved from https://fetchacure.org/pen-pals/.

Frank, G. (1984). The Boulder model: History, rationale, and critique. *Professional Psychology: Research and Practice, 15*(3), 417–435.

Friedmann, E., Katcher, A. H., Lynch, J. J., & Thomas, S. A. (1980). Animal companions and one-year survival of patients after discharge from a coronary care unit. *Public Health Reports, 95*(4), 307.

Griffin, J. A., McCune, S., Maholmes, V., & Hurley, K. (2011). Human-animal interaction research: An introduction to issues and topics. In L. Marston (Ed.), *How animals affect us: Examining the influence of human–animal interaction on child development and human health* (pp. 3–9).

Grinker, R. R., Sr. (1979). *Fifty years in psychiatry: A living history*. Springfield, IL: Charles C. Thomas.

Harris, M. D., Rinehart, J. M., & Gerstman, J. (1993). Animal-assisted therapy for the homebound elderly. *Holistic Nursing Practice, 8*(1), 27–37.

Hines, L. M. (2003). Historical perspectives on the human-animal bond. *American Behavioral Scientist, 47*(1), 7–15.

Hooker, S. D., Freeman, L. H., & Stewart, P. (2002). Pet therapy research: A historical review. *Holistic Nursing Practice, 17*(1), 17–23.

Klontz, B. T., Bivens, A., Leinart, D, & Klontz, T. (2007). The effectiveness of equine-assisted experiential therapy: Results of an open clinical trial. *Society & Animals, 15*, 257–267.

Levinson, B. M. (1962). The dog as a "co-therapist". *Mental Hygiene, 46*, 59–65.

Levinson, B. M. (1969). *Pet-oriented child psychotherapy*. Springfield, IL: Thomas.

Levinson, B. M. (1978). Pets and personality development. *Psychological Reports, 42*, 1031–1038.

McCardle, P., McCune, S., Netting, F. E., Berger, A., & Maholmes, V. (2011). In therapeutic human–animal interaction: An overview. In P. McCardle, S. McCune, J. Griffin, L. Esposito, & L. Freund (Eds.), *Animals in our lives. Human–animal interaction in family, community and therapeutic settings* (pp. 107–115). Baltimore, MA: Paul H. Brookes Publishing.

Nightingale, F. (1860). *Notes on nursing. New York: Dover 1967 NIH. (1988). The health benefits of pets.* Summary of workshop held 10–11 Sept. 1987, National Institutes of Health, Office of Medical Applications of Research (DHHS Publication No. 88-216-107). Washington, DC: US Government Printing Office, Bethesda, MD.

Serpell, J. A. (2011). Historical and cultural perspectives on human-pet interactions. In*Animals in our lives. Human–animal interaction in family, community and therapeutic settings* (pp. 11–22). Baltimore, MA: Paul H. Brookes Publishing.

Tuke, S. (1813). *Description of the retreat, an institution near York, for insane persons of the society of friends.* London: (n.p.).

CHAPTER 2

Human–Animal Interaction Analysis

Abstract At some level, animal-assisted intervention (AAI) involves humans interacting with animals. However, it is unknown which kinds of interactions occur between humans and animals during interventions and which interactions, if any, elicit specific outcomes. Human–animal interaction (HAI) is studied as a construct affecting human health and well-being, without a clear understanding of its critical components. This chapter argues for analysis of HAI as a process variable in AAI. The Human–Animal Interaction Scale (HAIS) is introduced as a way of gathering behavioral interaction data to study intervention processes. Following a discussion of instrument development and validation, research is reviewed to demonstrate HAI analysis.

Keywords Measurement • Instrumentation • Human–animal interaction • HAI analysis

Measurement

Measurement is defined as the assignment of scores to represent some characteristic (Price et al. 2017), such as measuring potential energy in physics or determining internal temperature when cooking food. Referring back to Chap. 1, clinicians and researchers have been measuring and recording animal-assisted intervention (AAI) outcomes through formal research since the 1960s (Hooker et al. 2002). Measurement within the

A. K. Fournier, *Animal-Assisted Intervention*,
https://doi.org/10.1007/978-3-030-32972-3_2

field of AAI often involves measuring psychological variables. Potential outcomes include, but are not limited to, psychological symptoms (e.g., improvements in depression, anxiety), psychosocial constructs (e.g., shifts in self-esteem, self-efficacy), attitudes, beliefs, and observable behavior. Many of the variables measured are internal factors that cannot be observed directly (e.g., attitude, beliefs). Psychometrics is the branch in psychology concerned with measurement of mental attributes, behavior, and performance (American Psychological Association 2018). AAI evaluation and research involves measuring all of these to varying degrees.

Animal-Assisted Intervention Measurement

Measurement of AAI outcomes can include self-report measures, physiological measures, or behavioral observations. For example, clients might complete a self-report of experiences or symptoms before and after treatment that involves an animal. Pendry et al. (2018) did this when evaluating an animal-assisted stress reduction program for college students. The students completed a self-report instrument rating their emotions before and after spending time with a shelter animal. Contentment was higher and anxiety was lower after the intervention. Regarding physiological measures, several studies have found reductions in cortisol, a hormonal marker for stress, following interactions with dogs (e.g., Barker et al. 2005; Odendaal 2000; Odendaal and Meintjes 2003; Viau et al. 2010). As an example of behavioral measures, Richeson (2003) studied the effects of an animal-assisted therapeutic recreation intervention on agitated behavior in adults with dementia. Agitated behaviors were significantly lower at posttest. Note that this study, like many others, addressed behavioral *outcomes* but not the actual behaviors occurring during the intervention. This is not surprising, as research on AAI has focused more on outcomes in general, and less on underlying processes and mechanisms of change. Rigorous outcome research is certainly important; we need to know whether AAI can result in reliable outcomes. In addition, we need to know how or why those outcomes come about. And beyond that, we need to understand whether the outcomes can be tied to the *animal(s)*. What, if anything, does HAI have to do with it? This is an important aspect of thinking empirically about AAI, addressed throughout the book.

Measuring Human–Animal Interaction

At the most basic level, AAI involves humans interacting with animals. HAI is an umbrella term to describe the wide array of interactions that occur between humans and nonhuman animals. The American Veterinary Medical Association (AVMA) defines HAI as any situation where there is interchange between human(s) and animal(s) at an individual or cultural level (AVMA 2019). The literature on HAI has grown in the last decade, with a major focus on the *effects* of HAI on human health and well-being and less focus on HAI itself.

For example, Pedersen et al. (2012) conducted a randomized controlled trial (RCT) on green care for depression. Green care is an intervention in which nature and the natural environment are used to promote health and well-being (Sempik et al. 2010); the intervention often includes working on a farm and caring for farm animals (e.g., Ross 2011). Pedersen and colleagues measured depression, anxiety, and self-efficacy before and after a 12-week intervention. Both depression and self-efficacy improved, compared to a wait-list control. Authors speculated on potential explanations for the improvements, including social support provided by the farm animals. However, data were not collected on what that social support entailed. For instance, did the animals make eye contact with or approach participants? In what ways, if any, did the participants engage with the animals that could have been experienced as social support? The authors provide examples of ***potential*** interactions. When describing a session in which participants worked with a farmer in the cowshed, they state that "participants were allowed to choose work such as grooming, mucking, feeding, taking care of the calves, and milking" (Pedersen et al. 2012, p. 153). This description of potential behavior is helpful in picturing behavioral aspects of the intervention, and consistent with AAI reporting in general. Still, it is unknown which of these behaviors occurred and whether they had an impact on participant outcomes. Analysis of behavioral interactions between humans and animals is critical to understanding AAI.

In Chap. 1, I shared how my interests in AAI began by studying prison-based dog programs. My dissertation research assessed the PenPals program (FETCH a Cure 2018) at a medium-security prison in the southeastern US. Inmates were educated in dog-training skills and worked in teams to care for and train shelter dogs in basic obedience. After several weeks of training in prison, the dogs graduated and were adopted by individuals and families in the community. In studying the program, I was curious about how much the inmates were able to interact with the dogs and whether differential amounts of interaction were related to outcomes. To my surprise there were no instruments available to quantify interaction between humans and animals.

Instrumentation

Because AAI research has focused on outcomes for human health and well-being, research to date has largely addressed measuring psychological constructs. Studies have used instruments that might be used to measure outcomes of psychological interventions in general (e.g., human thoughts, feelings, attitudes, beliefs, and behaviors). In addition, there is a growing list of animal-related measures designed to examine the human–animal bond and variables important to AAI. For example, there are instruments to measure the emotional attachment one has to their pets, such as the Companion Animal Bonding Scale (Poresky et al. 1987) or the Lexington Attachment to Pets Scale (Johnson et al. 1992). Other instruments measure attitudes toward animals, such as the Pet Attitude Scale (Templer et al. 2004; Templer et al. 1981). There are quite a few instruments addressing the costs and benefits of pet keeping, including the Dog Care Responsibility Inventory (Davis 1987) and the Pet Expectations Inventory (Kidd et al. 1992). See Anderson (2007) for a compendium of these and other measures related to the human–animal bond. In addition, Herzog and Dorr (2000) compiled a list of surveys specific to attitudes toward animals.

Unfortunately, none of these instruments could help in the examination of the kind and quantity of interactions happening between inmates and dogs at the prison. Necessity being the mother of invention, I created a self-report measure for inmates to rate their level of interaction with the dogs. With the help of colleagues and students, this has become the Human–Animal Interaction Scale (HAIS). Using it in AAI practice and research has fueled a passion to understand the *what* (what is happening) and stimulated ideas for investigating the *how* (how do animals help human health).

Measuring any variable, whether measuring symptoms in clients to determine treatment progress or measuring variables in research to test an intervention, requires an effective instrument. Instruments used to measure psychosocial constructs are evaluated on two broad features: reliability and validity. A reliable instrument measures accurately and is consistent; a valid instrument measures what it is intended to measure. An in-depth discussion of these features is beyond the scope of this book, but the reader can learn more about psychometrics in general from any number of sources on psychological testing (e.g., Kaplan and Saccuzzo 2017). More specific to AAI, Wilson and Netting (2012) reviewed the status of instruments in the HAI field. They provide a review of psychometric concepts, identify shortcomings of existing measures, and give suggestions for developing new instruments. As an example of the steps taken in instrument development, and to encourage measurement of HAI specifically, I next provide information on development of the HAIS.

Human–Animal Interaction Scale

The HAIS is a self-report instrument designed to describe and quantify behavioral interactions between humans and animals. The scale allows for (1) standardized description of interactions that occur between humans and animals and (2) quantification of overall interaction within a distinct period of time. The HAIS lists 24 behaviors that can be emitted from a human toward an animal (e.g., *watch*, *pet*, *groom*) or from an animal toward a human (e.g., *sniff*, *lick*, *make friendly sounds*). After a period of interaction with an animal, respondents rate the extent to which each behavior occurred on a scale from 0 (not at all) to 4 (a great deal). Item ratings sum for totals of human-initiated and animal-initiated behavior; these subtotals are summed for a total score indicating an overall quantity of HAI.[1]

Scale Development

I include a brief summary of the scale's development and validation here. For a more detailed description, see Fournier et al. (2016). The HAIS was developed by reviewing the HAI literature, observing AAI, and interviewing AAI practitioners. From this, items were written to reflect the range of behaviors that could occur when humans and animals are interacting. An initial list of items was tested in the laboratory with college students. Volunteer research participants spent brief, unstructured time with an animal and then responded to the items. In addition to participant report,

[1] A copy of the HAIS is provided in Appendix A.

researchers observed the interactions and rated the same items. Items were added, deleted, or revised based on these data. Once the list of items was finalized, the scale was administered to research participants in a variety of settings to determine its psychometric properties.

Reliability and Validity

Development and validation of a psychological test or measurement instrument involves evaluating the test for reliability and validity. The process entails gathering various types of evidence via multiple calculations and comparisons. Table 2.1 provides a list of terms, the accompanying statistic, and the evidence-gathering method used in development of the HAIS.

Internal consistency of an instrument is the degree to which it measures the same construct throughout. This was determined by calculating Cronbach's alpha on HAIS scores from participants in multiple settings. Alpha scores indicated the HAIS was internally consistent with inmates in the PenPals prison-based dog program ($\alpha = 0.86$, $n = 132$), university students reporting on HAI in the past six months ($\alpha = 0.89$, $n = 41$), university students interacting with animals in a laboratory ($\alpha = 0.76$, $n = 57$), and clients participating in equine-assisted learning ($\alpha = 0.72$, $n = 65$). Regarding different species, data indicated the scale was internally

Table 2.1 Psychometric terms, definitions, and examples

Psychometric property	*Definition*	*Example evidence for the HAIS*
Reliability		
Internal consistency	Instrument measures the same construct throughout	Cronbach's alpha calculated on HAIS scores across settings
Test–retest reliability	Scores remain the same when administered at two different times	Correlation between HAIS scores at time 1 (after session) and time 2 (one week later)
Validity		
Convergent validity	Scores on the developing measure are similar to scores on other measures of the same construct	Correlation between scores on the HAIS and the Companion Animal Bonding Scale
Discriminant validity	Scores on the new measure are different from scores on measures of different constructs	Correlation between HAIS scores and the Companion Animal Semantic Differential

consistent when measuring HAI with cats and dogs ($\alpha = 0.84$, $n = 157$), small mammals like rabbits and rats ($\alpha = 0.74$, $n = 32$), and horses ($\alpha = 0.72$, $n = 65$).

Test–retest reliability evaluates the error associated with administering a test at two different times (Kaplan and Saccuzzo 2017). It is an estimate of the instrument's ability to give the same results, given the construct has not changed. The HAIS test–retest reliability was examined with college students interacting with companion animals in a laboratory setting. The students interacted with animals, completed the HAIS immediately, and then returned to complete the HAIS again one week later. The correlation between the two administrations was acceptable, $r = 0.70$–0.94.

There are several different types of evidence for an instrument's validity; together they help estimate whether the instrument measures what it is designed to measure. Evidence for construct validity can come from several different types of validity, including convergent and discriminant. Convergent validity is demonstrated when scores on the developing measure converge or are similar to scores on other measures of the same construct. A comparison of the HAIS with the Companion Animal Bonding Scale (Poresky et al. 1987) provided evidence of convergent validity ($r = 0.38$, $p = 0.004$). Discriminant validity is the extent to which scores on the new measure are different from scores on measures of different constructs. In other words, the question is whether the instrument can discriminate between the construct of interest and some other construct. Evidence for discriminant validity was provided by comparisons between the HAIS and the Companion Animal Semantic Differential (CASD) (Poresky et al. 1988). The CASD is a set of adjectives set on a semantic differential; respondents are asked to rate a childhood pet on each of the adjectives. The score provides an estimate of one's bond with a pet, a construct quite different from behavioral HAI occurring with an unfamiliar animal at a distinct point in time. As we expected, HAIS scores did not correlate with scores on this scale, showing discrimination between our construct of interest and other constructs related to the human–animal bond ($r = 0.16$, $p = 0.233$).

Human–Animal Interaction Analysis

The HAIS is unique in that it is designed to describe and quantify the actual interactions that occur during AAI, allowing for an analysis of behavior within an intervention. My research team and I have used the HAIS in various capacities. Data from two different studies are shared here to illustrate utility of HAI analysis in studying HAI as a basic phenomenon and an AAI process variable. The studies involve analyzing HAI in (1) a laboratory study with college students and (2) a correlational study with a clinical sample.

HAI Analysis in the Laboratory

We conducted a study to examine HAI in a laboratory setting, with a non-clinical sample of 57 college students. The students volunteered to participate in research in exchange for extra credit in an undergraduate psychology course. Participants reported to the laboratory, completed informed consent, and spent three minutes of unstructured time with an animal. The animal was either a companion animal (i.e., cat or dog; $n = 25$) or a small mammal (i.e., rabbit, rat, or hedgehog; $n = 32$). More specifically, participants were brought to an observation room with the animal and invited to "*interact as little or as much as you like.*"[2]

Figure 2.1 is a bar graph showing mean ratings for human-initiated behaviors emitted toward the animal. The data are separated by species category, showing similarities and differences in the students' behavior toward companion animals and small mammals. These data are typical of all the research we have done with the HAIS in that a variety of behaviors were indicated, with some rated higher than others.

I show these data not to suggest that all humans will emit these behaviors toward animals in these ratios. This is one small sample of college students in one particular laboratory with several specific animals. Instead, this is an example of the kind of data we can collect to better understand AAI. In addition to measuring therapeutic outcomes like mood or functioning pre and post, we can examine which particular behaviors occur. While these data are intended to serve as an example and not define HAI, they are consistent with several other studies our team has conducted. We tend to see some behaviors rated much higher (i.e., *watch*, *spend time near*, *pet*, *talk*) than other behaviors (i.e., *hug*, *kiss*, *hold*). Taking pictures or videos of the animal tends to be rated very low. This is inconsistent with our society's current practice of taking numerous pictures and sharing on social media (e.g., Bányai et al. 2017). Some people have even been in danger because of their desire for a media-worthy selfie with animals in a zoo or in the wild (e.g., Bever 2019; Daly 2019). However, participants

[2] During the unstructured interaction, researchers observed from outside the room via a one-way mirrored window and intercom and were trained to interrupt at any signs of harm or distress to the humans or animals.

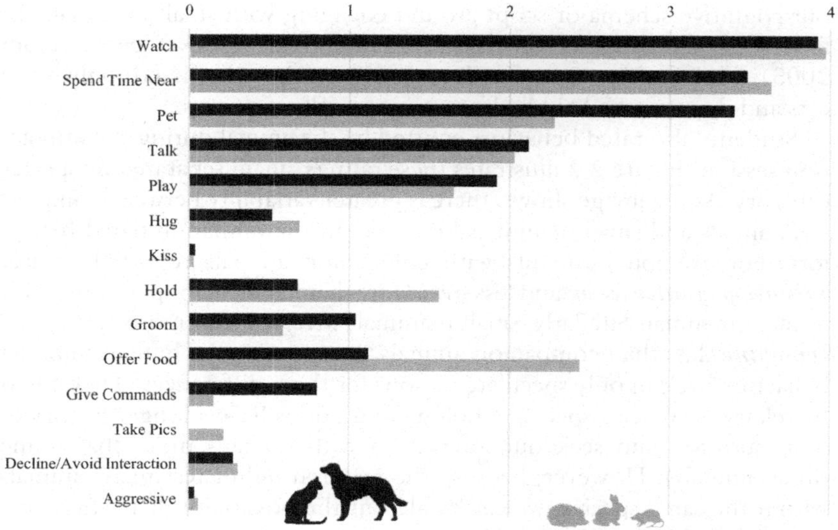

Fig. 2.1 Human-initiated interaction with companion animals versus small mammals. The figure depicts behaviors university students emitted toward companion animals (i.e., cat or dog) and small mammals (i.e., rabbit, rat, or hedgehog)

in the present study were students volunteering for extra credit in a class, and the research took place within the psychology department on campus. It may be that participants were still within their role as students in an academic setting and thus phone use followed perceived classroom norms (e.g., no phone use allowed).

Research like this could be important in better understanding how HAI differs by species. In this sample, we see that there are many similarities between the way students acted toward companion animals and small mammals. Ratings are similar for *watch*, *spend time near*, *pet*, *talk*, *play*, *hug*, and *kiss*. There are also important differences; *hold* and *offer food* were rated much higher for small mammals than companion animals. Although the observation room always contained toys and treats specific to the animal present, you can see that small mammals were offered food more often than companion animals. On the other hand, small mammals were not *given commands* for tricks or training as often as companion animals were. We can only speculate on reasons for these differences. For example, holding a rat or hedgehog may be more feasible and more consistent with our cognitive schema or script around engaging with small mammals. In fact, these animals are sometimes referred to as "pocket pets" (Flom 2005), implying they are animals to hold. On the other hand, only some cats and dogs can be held by humans, especially strangers.

Students also rated behaviors emitted by the animal during the interaction session. Figure 2.2 illustrates these ratings, again separated by species category. As the image shows, there is greater variability between companion animals and small mammals here than in the human-initiated behaviors. For example, students with companion animals reported greater *initiation of interaction* and less *avoidance* than those who spent time with a small mammal. Similarly, small mammals *accepted food* more and *obeyed commands* less than companion animals. Just as with the human-initiated behaviors, we can only speculate reasons for these differences. They could be related to species-specific ethology (e.g., dogs have a longer history of domestication and seek out interaction with humans more than some other animals). However, because the research didn't test many animals within the same species, we can't rule out the possibility that differences reflect individual variation within the species. Again, this provides an example of the kinds of data that can be gathered to better understand AAI and its active components.

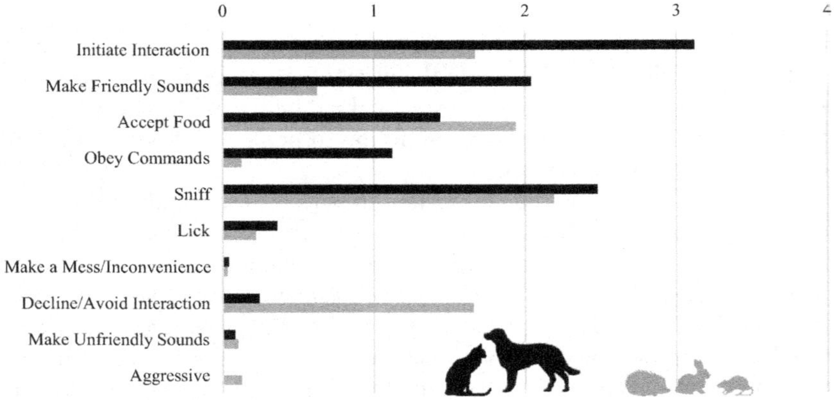

Fig. 2.2 Animal-initiated interaction with companion animals versus small mammals. The graph shows behaviors emitted by animals toward students. Animals are separated into species categories—companion animals (i.e., cat or dog) and small mammals (i.e., rabbit, rat, or hedgehog)

In thinking empirically about behavioral HAI, we might wonder whether behaviors emitted by humans and animals differ by species. Figure 2.3 shows the quantity of human- and animal-initiated behavior for each individual species tested. As the figure shows, the amount of human-initiated interaction did not differ for this sample, regardless of which animal was involved. However, animal-initiated behavior did differ. According to the student participants, dogs emitted more interactive behaviors ($M = 13.47$, $SD = 5.12$) than the hedgehog ($M = 6.80$, $SD = 4.66$), rat ($M = 5.96$, $SD = 4.74$), and rabbit ($M = 4.33$, $SD = 5.69$). These differences were statistically significant, $F(4, 51) = 6.84$, $p < 0.001$.

These are self-report data, in which students rated the degree to which they and the animal engaged in interactive behaviors. In addition, *researchers* watched the sessions and completed the HAIS based on their *observations*. Findings were similar; dogs *initiated interaction* more than each of the other animals, $F(4, 52) = 3.55$, $p = 0.012$. Overall, these data suggest that students and animals engaged in a range of behaviors and there were identifiable differences in animal behavior between dogs and other species. Next, I'll describe the HAI we have analyzed in a more applied setting—equine-assisted psychotherapy and learning (EAP).

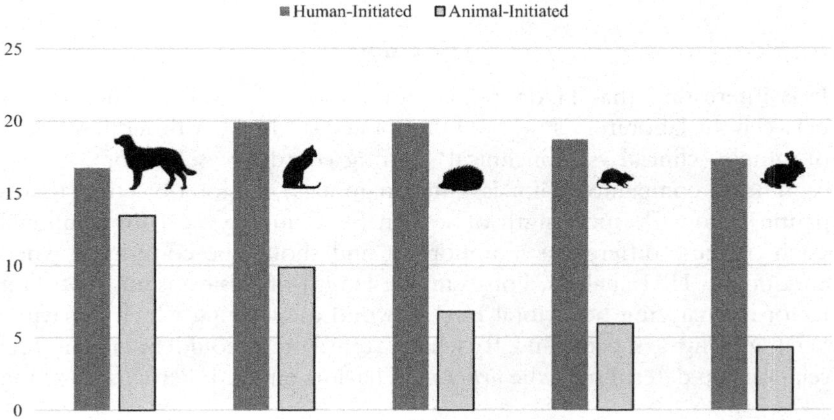

Fig. 2.3 Human–animal interaction across species. Graph showing the quantity of human- and animal-initiated interactions for several species, as reported on the HAIS. Species, from left to right, are dog, cat, hedgehog, rat, and rabbit

HAI Analysis in an Applied Setting

A correlational study was conducted to explore HAI as it occurs during sessions at a local private-practice counseling center that provides EAP. Most clients at the practice complete the HAIS after EAP sessions. The scores are entered into a client database that is de-identified for research purposes. The data reported here are from 100 EAP clients attending an individual or group EAP session. Sessions last 60–90 minutes, occur in an outdoor pasture or indoor horse arena, and follow the Equine-Assisted Growth and Learning Association (Eagala) model[3] (Eagala 2015). Participants completed the HAIS form immediately following the session, reporting on their interactions with the horses.

Figure 2.4 shows human- and animal-initiated behaviors. Consistent with the laboratory study, EAP clients reported a range of behaviors. Each of the items on the scale were endorsed to some degree, with some being rated much higher than others. The highest-rated human behaviors were *spending time near*, *watching*, and *petting* the horses. This is consistent with ratings for both companion animals and small mammals in the laboratory study. Similarly, the highest-rated animal behaviors were *initiate interaction*, *sniff*, and *make friendly sounds*. These were also the highest-rated behaviors in the laboratory, across both companion animals and small mammals.

Discussion

It is interesting that HAIS ratings are so similar given the differences between the laboratory study and the applied study. They differ in the type of sample (clinical vs. nonclinical), setting (outdoor vs. indoor), species (equine vs. companion animals/small mammals), session objective (therapeutic vs. open), and length of session (4 minutes vs. 60–90 minutes). Each of these differences is important and should be considered when conducting HAI analysis. For example, length of session is an important factor in analyzing behavioral HAI. Beyond cataloguing which behaviors occur during a session and to what extent, there could be a temporal relationship determining the *order* of behaviors emitted. Perhaps watching

[3] Sessions within this model are facilitated by a licensed mental health professional and equine specialist, are ground-based (no riding), are solution-oriented, and follow the Eagala code of ethics.

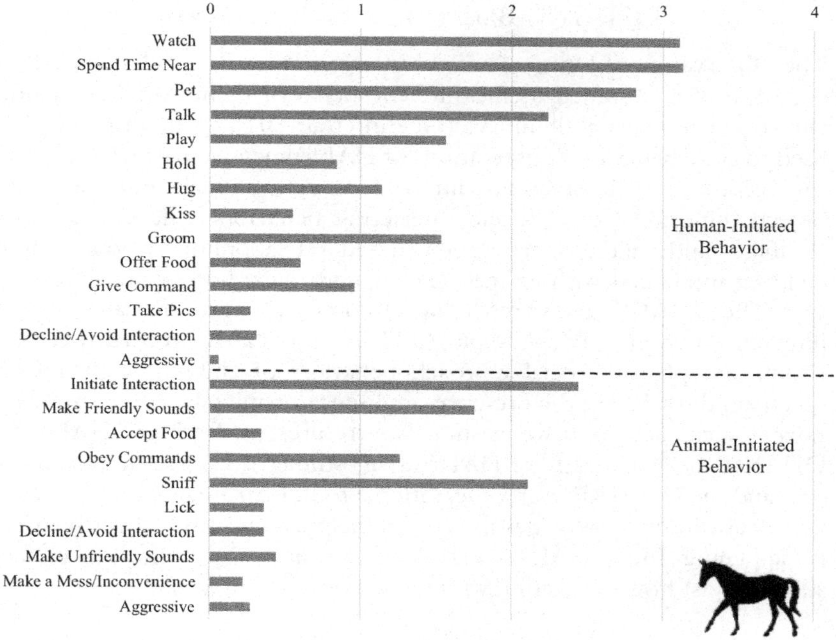

Fig. 2.4 HAI in equine-assisted psychotherapy and learning. The graph shows the variation in behavioral interactions reported by clients following an equine-assisted psychotherapy or learning session

the animal occurs first, then the human moves near to them, then pets them, then talks to them. If this were the case, the session would need to last long enough to get through the chain of behaviors in order to reach the point of talking to the animal. Maybe this could happen in 4 minutes but there is a greater (although not guaranteed) chance of it happening within 60–90 minutes. Therefore, the length of the session could determine which behaviors occur, rather than some personal factor within the human or animal, or some relationship developing between them. Examining HAI through self-report on the HAIS is just one aspect of HAI analysis. Coding observational data provides additional information for illuminating the HAI within AAI.

OHAIRE Behavioral Coding Tool

The Observation of Human–Animal Interaction for Research (OHAIRE) coding tool is designed to measure the behavior of humans interacting with other humans and animals (Guérin et al. 2018). The instrument is used to code behavioral observations of HAI from video data. Researchers can record social interactions, interactions with animals and inanimate objects, emotional display, and interfering behaviors. The instrument's reliability and validity were demonstrated via laboratory studies where children interacted with animals (i.e., guinea pigs, horses, and dogs) or toys. The OHAIRE allows researchers to observe and record categories of interactive behavior. For example, O'Haire et al. (2013) recorded verbal, visual, and physical social-approach behaviors of children with autism spectrum disorders in the presence or absence of animals. Results showed greater social approach when animals were present. Both the HAIS and OHAIRE provide means for HAI analysis—the HAIS as a self-report measure and the OHAIRE as an observational tool. Instruments such as these, as well as those yet to be developed, can help us objectively describe what is happening during AAI. That kind of HAI analysis is critical to understanding just how interacting with animals affects humans.

Summary

The goal of this chapter was to discuss measurement as an important issue in thinking empirically about AAI. After defining the concept and discussing the state of instruments in the field, the HAIS was introduced as a self-report measure to describe and quantify interaction between humans and animals. HAI analysis was illustrated with laboratory-based and applied data, comparing interaction behavior across species and settings. The interactions between humans and animals shown here should not be interpreted as definitive of species- or setting-specific behavior. Behavioral HAI can be affected by a variety of factors, including human/animal temperament, learning history, or a complex interaction between variables specific to the human, the animal, and the situation. Drawing definitive conclusions requires testing with larger, more diverse samples. The utility of sharing them here is to illustrate the importance of and potential for conducting HAI analysis to better understand AAI.

Seeing the variety of interactions that occur during research or intervention sessions has spurred more questions about AAI for our research team. For example, do these differing levels of behavior represent different *doses* of HAI? Furthermore, does HAI *dose* impact AAI outcome? This concept of dose is discussed in Chap. 3.

References

American Psychological Association. (2018). *Psychometrics*. APA dictionary of psychology. Retrieved from https://dictionary.apa.org/psychometrics.

American Veterinary Medical Association. (2019). The human-animal interaction and human-animal bond. Retrieved from https://www.avma.org/KB/Policies/Pages/The-Human-Animal-Bond.aspx.

Anderson, D. C. (2007). Assessing the human-animal bond: A compendium of actual measures. In A. M. Beck (Ed.), *New directions in the human-animal bond series*. West Lafayette, IN: Purdue University Press.

Bányai, F., Zsila, Á., Király, O., Maraz, A., Elekes, Z., Griffiths, M. D., et al. (2017). Problematic social media use: Results from a large-scale nationally representative adolescent sample. *PLoS One, 12*(1), e0169839.

Barker, S. B., Knisely, J. S., McCain, N. L., & Best, A. M. (2005). Measuring stress and immune responses in health care professionals following interaction with a therapy dog: A pilot study. *Psychological Reports, 96*, 713–729.

Bever, L. (2019, March 10). A woman was trying to take a selfie with a jaguar when it attached her, authorities say. *The Washington Post*. Retrieved from https://www.washingtonpost.com/science/2019/03/10/woman-was-trying-take-selfie-with-jaguar-when-it-attacked-her-authorities-say/?utm_term=.e37de1314bd6.

Daly, N. (2019, March 12). Why people risk their lives for the ultimate animal selfie. *National Geographic*. Retrieved from https://www.nationalgeographic.com/animals/2019/03/psychology-of-why-people-enter-wild-animal-enclosures-at-zoos/.

Davis, J. H. (1987). Pet care during preadolescence: Development considerations. *Child: Care, Health and Development, 139*(4), 269–276.

Equine Assisted Growth and Learning Association. (2015). *Fundamentals of the EAGALA model: Practice untraining manual* (8th ed.). Santaquin, UT: EAGALA.

FETCH a Cure. (2018). *Pen Pals*. Retrieved from https://fetchacure.org/pen-pals/.

Flom, B. L. (2005). Counseling with pocket pets: Using small animals in elementary counseling programs. *Professional School Counseling, 8*, 469–471.

Fournier, A. K., Berry, T. D., Letson, E. E., & Chanen, R. (2016). The human-animal interaction scale: Development and evaluation. *Anthrozoös, 29*(3), 455–467.

Guérin, N. A., Gabriels, R. L., Germone, M. M., Schuck, S. E., Traynor, A., Thomas, K. M., et al. (2018). Reliability and validity assessment of the observation of human-animal interaction for research (OHAIRE) behavior coding tool. *Frontiers in Veterinary Science, 5*. https://doi.org/10.3389/fvets.2018.00268.

Herzog, H., & Dorr, L. (2000). Electronically available surveys of attitudes toward animals. *Society & Animals, 8*(2), 183–190.

Hooker, S. D., Freeman, L. H., & Stewart, P. (2002). Pet therapy research: A historical review. *Holistic Nursing Practice, 17*(1), 17–23.

Johnson, T. P., Garrity, T. F., & Stallones, L. (1992). Psychometric evaluation of the Lexington attachment to pets scale (LAPS). *Anthrozoös, 5*(3), 160–175.

Kaplan, R. M., & Saccuzzo, D. P. (2017). *Psychological testing: Principles, applications, and issues* (9th ed.). Boston, MA: Cengage.

Kidd, A. H., Kidd, R. M., & George, C. C. (1992). Veterinarians and successful pet adoptions. *Psychological Reports, 71*, 551–557.

O'Haire, M. E., McKenzie, S. J., Beck, A. M., & Slaughter, V. (2013). Social behaviors increase in children with autism in the presence of animals compared to toys. *PLoS One, 8*(2), e57010. https://doi.org/10.1371/journal.pone.0057010.

Odendaal, J. S. (2000). Animal-assisted therapy—Magic or medicine? *Journal of Psychosomatic Research, 49*, 275–280.

Odendaal, J. S., & Meintjes, R. A. (2003). Neurophysiological correlates of affiliative behavior between humans and dogs. *Veterinary Journal, 165*, 296–301.

Pedersen, I., Martinsen, E. W., Berget, B., & Braastad, B. O. (2012). Farm animal-assisted intervention for people with clinical depression: A randomized controlled trial. *Anthrozoös, 25*(2), 149–160.

Pendry, P., Carr, A. M., Roeter, S. M., & Vandagriff, J. L. (2018). Experimental trial demonstrates effects of animal-assisted stress prevention program on college students' positive and negative emotion. *Human-Animal Interaction Bulletin, 6*(1), 81–97.

Poresky, R. H., Hendrix, C., Mosier, J. E., & Samuelson, M. L. (1987). The companion animal bonding scale: Internal reliability and construct validity. *Psychological Reports, 60*(3), 743–746.

Poresky, R. H., Hendrix, C., Mosier, J. E., & Samuelson, M. L. (1988). The companion animal semantic differential: Long and short form reliability and validity. *Educational and Psychological Measurement, 48*(1), 255–260.

Price, P. C., Jhangiani, R., Chiang, I. A., Leighton, D. C., & Cuttler, C. (2017). *Research methods in psychology*, 3rd American edition. Retrieved from https://open.umn.edu/opentextbooks/textbooks/research-methods-in-psychology-3rd-american-edition.

Richeson, N. E. (2003). Effects of animal-assisted therapy on agitated behaviors and social interactions of older adults with dementia. *American Journal of Alzheimer's Disease & Other Dementias, 18*(6), 353–358.

Ross, S. B. (2011). *The extraordinary spirit of green chimneys: Connecting children and animals to create hope*. West Lafayette, IN: Purdue University Press.

Sempik, J., Hine, R., & Wilcox, D. (2010). Green care: A conceptual framework. A report of the working group on the health benefits of green care. In *COST 866, green care in agriculture*. Loughborough: Loughborough University.

Templer, D. I., Salter, C. A., Dickey, S., Baldwin, R., & Veleber, D. M. (1981). The construction of a pet attitude scale. *The Psychological Record, 31*(3), 343–348.

Templer, D., Arikawa, H., Canfield, M., Munsell, K., & Tangan, K. (2004). Modification of the pet attitude scale. *Society & Animals, 12*(2), 137–142.

Viau, R., Arsenault-Lapierre, G., Fecteau, S., Champagne, N., Walker, C.-D., & Lupien, S. (2010). Effect of service dogs on salivary cortisol secretion in autistic children. *Psychoneuroendocrinology, 35*(8), 1187.

Wilson, C. C., & Netting, F. E. (2012). The status of instrument development in the human–animal interaction field. *Anthrozoös, 25*, 11–55.

CHAPTER 3

HAI Dose in Animal-Assisted Intervention

Abstract This chapter identifies human–animal interaction (HAI) dose as a construct of study for animal-assisted intervention (AAI) practice and research. To date, AAI studies have defined dose similarly to studies on traditional psychotherapy—number of sessions, length of sessions, and length of treatment. A case is made for studying intervention components separately, including HAI dose. Two studies are described, examining these dose–effect relationships. Dose–response curves are shown to illustrate the nature of the relationship between HAI and outcomes. In both a laboratory study and an applied study, defining dose by self-report scores and time spent respectively, the relationship appears to be nonlinear. Dose–response curves were hyperbolic, with a period of exponential growth followed by a plateau. The findings suggest the dose–response relationship for HAI and distress is more complex than "the more the merrier."

Keywords Human–animal interaction • Dose • Medical model • Dose–response relationship

Thinking empirically about animal-assisted intervention (AAI) includes being curious about the process. As practitioners and researchers, we must wonder what's happening, is it working, and if so how? I'm curious about all of these questions. Using the medical model may be helpful in organizing findings, putting vague stories and descriptions into more objective

A. K. Fournier, *Animal-Assisted Intervention*,
https://doi.org/10.1007/978-3-030-32972-3_3

clinical terms, and developing testable research questions. The medical model is certainly not the only way to think about AAI or other interventions. But it is the system within which many practitioners and clients find themselves.

Research tends to imply animals are an active ingredient in the AAI process. In other words, the animal has some effect. For example, pioneering research by Friedman and colleagues (1980) found the survival rate following myocardial infarction or angina was higher for people with pets than those without pets. Although not examined in the study, authors speculated that pets benefit patients by providing and being a target for attention, as well as providing contact comfort. Crossman (2017) conducted a systematic review of the literature on HAI. Results showed a small-to-medium effect size for distress reduction (e.g., mood/affect, depression, anxiety), but a lack of evidence to attribute effects to the animal. The author calls for rigorous research to investigate the "black box" of HAI, examining the how and why of HAI-related distress reduction (Crossman 2017, p. 11). One way to examine explanatory mechanisms is to apply the medical model, as it is used to determine effects of other treatments such as medicines and other physical interventions. For example, when a new medication is developed, what are the questions that must be answered and how do researchers go about answering them? The remainder of this chapter addresses just one of these issues—*dose*—as it may apply to AAI.

Animal-Assisted Intervention Dose

The Merriam-Webster dictionary defines *dose* as the measured quantity of a therapeutic agent to be taken at one time (2019). In terms of AAI, the therapeutic agent could be the intervention as a whole, or there could be multiple components within the intervention that serve as therapeutic agents. Major components within an AAI could be a therapy program or curriculum (e.g., manualized anger management program), a human practitioner (e.g., animal handler, psychotherapist, educator, etc.), and one or more therapy animals. Research articles on AAI tend to discuss the intervention as a whole. As mentioned earlier, clients who receive an AAI are studied at pre and post or compared to clients who receive an intervention without animals. Regarding dose, authors are most likely to describe the number of AAI sessions attended, length of sessions, and topic covered.

Session Duration and Frequency

Kamioka et al. (2014) conducted a systematic review of randomized controlled trials (RCTs) on AAI. They found 11 studies meeting RCT criteria, 7 of which investigated mental health–related variables. The treatments tested included a wide range of interactions between clients and animals. Across the studies, duration of session ranged from 15 minutes to 3 hours, length of intervention ranged from 1 day to 12 weeks, sessions ran from 1 to 3 times per week, and multiple animals were used (e.g., dogs, horses, dolphins, fish). Quality and quantity of interaction between humans and animals were not addressed; the focus of the research was outcomes. Variables related to dose (i.e., session length or frequency) were not discussed. However, the authors include intervention dose on a recommended research agenda to build AAI evidence.

Nimer and Lundahl's meta-analysis (2007) investigated whether the number of sessions reported in a study was related to the effect size. There were trends for a relationship between number of sessions and outcomes, but no significant correlations were found. A more recent meta-analysis on equine-assisted interventions for at-risk youth (Wilkie et al. 2016) found seven studies that met inclusion criteria. For those studies, AAI dose included weekly group sessions ranging from 50 minutes to 2 hours, running for an average of 5 to 12 weeks, but as long as 26 weeks. These studies resulted in moderate effect sizes when examining pre–post measures. The authors call for research to identify optimal treatment duration.

Jones et al. (2019) conducted a systematic review of research on canine-assisted psychotherapy. They found seven studies meeting inclusion criteria, with dose as one of the variables of study. Dose was defined as session frequency (i.e., once per week), session duration (ranging from 45 minutes to 3 hours per session), and length of treatment (ranging from 10 to 12 weeks). Dose was then calculated in hours by multiplying the duration of each session by the length of the treatment. Total hours ranged from 9 to 36 hours; the authors could not make conclusions on the role of dose in intervention outcomes. For each of these studies, dose was defined as frequency or duration of sessions or length of treatment and the intervention was tested as a whole, rather than examining different components within the intervention. Furthermore, none of the studies reviewed included an analysis of the interactions between humans and animals.

HAI Dose

HAI dose has not been thoroughly studied as of yet. Rather, studies treat it as an all-or-none variable; clients experience interaction with an animal or they don't. Experts in the field have expressed a need to explore the critical dose of HAI and its effects (Esposito et al. 2011; Serpell et al. 2017; Vitztum 2013). Although it was not discussed in the context of dose, the review by Jones et al. (2019) did address HAI. The authors categorized interaction with animals as spontaneous (client-led), structured (i.e., facilitator-led), or semi-structured. Of the seven studies reviewed, one included structured interaction, one included spontaneous interaction, and five included some combination of client- and facilitator-led interaction. While analyses did not test for relationships between the nature of the HAI and intervention outcome, the authors underscore the need for scholarly work around engagement with the animal(s) in AAI. Specifically, they call for a nomenclature to describe engagement with the animals and research to examine the outcomes of different types of engagement (i.e., interaction).

Research in environmental studies suggests increases in the presence of nature and biodiversity are associated with greater outcomes for human health and well-being. Fuller et al. (2007) studied the effect of varying degrees of species richness in urban green spaces. They measured species richness of plants, butterflies, and birds of various green spaces and surveyed visitors on their perceptions of the space and factors related to psychological well-being. Respondents in more species-rich habitats reported greater ability to think and gain perspective, a greater sense of identity from and connection with the green space, and greater emotional ties to the space. This was true for species richness of both plants and birds. The research suggests that varying the richness of nature present may vary psychological outcomes. Dallimer et al. (2012) conducted a similar study, with some conflicting findings. Participants' reported well-being was correlated with their *perceptions* of biodiversity, but not the *actual level* of biodiversity. This line of research measured plant- and animal-species richness, not HAI. Still, data suggest human well-being may be related to quantity of natural living things in the environment.

Cracknell et al. (2016) examined the effects of varying levels of aquarium-animal life, with dose defined as greater or lesser biodiversity. The researchers conducted a natural experiment, assessing patrons when a large aquarium was (a) filled with only seawater and artificial decoration,

(b) partially stocked with half the species and individual specimens of fish and crustaceans, and (c) fully stocked. Results showed higher rates of biodata were associated with greater time spent viewing, reduced heart rate, and better mood. The greatest differences were observed between the condition with no biodiversity and that with high biodiversity. Differences between low and high diversity were more mixed; reported mood was greater following the high dose but heart rate showed no difference. Looking at time spent viewing the aquarium, most gains in mood occurred within the first 5 minutes, with diminished returns from additional time spent. These data suggest dose may be defined by time spent or richness of stimuli in a natural environment. Each of these studies found tendencies toward greater outcomes with greater biodiversity of plants and animals. My students and I have examined dose in the context of HAI, with dose defined as self-reported quantity of interaction and time spent interacting. Next I share a laboratory study demonstrating (a) experimental manipulation of HAI dose and (b) a potential dose–response relationship between HAI and psychological state.

Experimental Manipulation of HAI Dose

An independent-groups experiment examined HAI dose in a laboratory by randomly assigning nonclinical college students to experience no HAI, a low dose of HAI, or a high dose of HAI. We hypothesized participants interacting with animals would report greater positive emotion than those in a no-HAI control group, and that the participants in the high-dose condition would report greater benefits than those in the low-dose condition. Participants were 75 college students who volunteered in exchange for extra credit in a psychology course. Students were recruited through class announcements and reported to the university laboratory. After completing informed consent, an individual participant would complete the Multidimensional Mood Scale (MDMS), a self-report instrument designed to measure mood state (Wilhelm and Schoebi 2007). Then they were randomly assigned to one of three conditions—a no-HAI control condition (2 minutes alone with reading materials), a low-dose HAI condition (2 minutes with a cat or dog), or a high-dose HAI condition (4 minutes with a cat or dog and species-specific toys, treats, and brushes). All participants were given the following instruction: "*This is 'Sweetie,' feel free to interact as little or as much as you like.*" After the designated time had elapsed, participants completed the MDMS (again) and the HAIS (Fournier et al. 2016), received an extra-credit slip, and were dismissed. At the conclusion of the study, students were debriefed with a classroom presentation.

To check whether HAI dose was manipulated, HAIS scores were compared between the low-dose HAI and high-dose HAI conditions. HAIS scores were significantly higher, meaning participants reported greater quantities of HAI in the high-dose condition ($M = 36.4$, SD = 10.6) than in the low-dose condition ($M = 27.4$, $SD = 7.8$), $F\ (1,\ 50) = 12.1$, $p = 0.001$. HAI dose, defined by HAIS scores, seemed to have been successfully manipulated.

Mood State Across HAI Dose Conditions

To determine whether mood differed across conditions, MDMS scores were first tested at pretest. The one-way ANOVA showed participants in all three groups were equal at pretest, $F\,(2,\ 74) = 0.918$, $p = 0.404$; we started with equivalent groups regarding mood. As Fig. 3.1 illustrates, the data were trending such that posttest mood increased with increasing HAI dose. An ANOVA indicated that posttest mood was significantly higher in

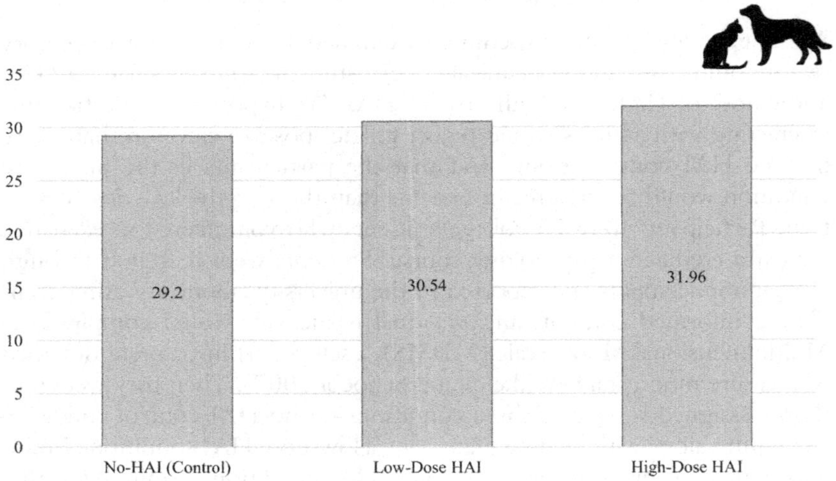

Fig. 3.1 Mood in no-, low-, and high-dose HAI conditions. Graph depicting the mean mood rating at posttest for 78 university students following unstructured interaction with a dog or cat. Mood was significantly higher in the high-dose condition than in the control condition, $F\,(2,\ 73) = 3.16$, $p = 0.048$

the high-dose condition ($M = 31.96$, $SD = 3.99$) than in the control condition ($M = 29.2$, $SD = 4.95$), $F(2, 73) = 3.16$, $p = 0.048$. However, post-test mood did not differ between the low-dose and control conditions ($p = 0.233$) nor between the low-dose and high-dose conditions ($p = 0.195$). Referring again to Fig. 3.1, only the conditions with the biggest difference in dose (control and high-dose) were significantly different. This is consistent with research by Cracknell et al. (2016), where aquarium visitors' positive feelings were greater in the fully stocked condition than in the unstocked condition, but there were no differences between the partially stocked and fully stocked conditions. These findings could be interpreted to mean that HAI is not dependent on dose; it is an all-or-none variable as it has been studied to date. Or, it could be that HAI dose matters but we didn't capture two distinct doses. Perhaps the critical dose is greater than the difference in HAI that can be captured in 2 versus 4 minutes, or between HAIS scores of 27 versus 36. For example, maybe a low dose of HAI is a HAIS score of 10 or less.

The MDMS measures three dimensions of mood: calm (i.e., tense vs. relaxed), valence (i.e., well vs. discontent), and energetic arousal (awake vs. fatigued) (Wilhelm and Schoebi 2007). An ANOVA was calculated to determine whether the difference in mood between the control and high-dose conditions was specific to one dimension or another. These individual dimensions did not differ between the conditions. As you can see in Fig. 3.2, the difference between the control and high-dose conditions cannot be attributed to any particular dimension of mood. Rather, there were small increases in each as dose increased; these small increases cumulated to an overall increase in mood with increased dose.

It should be noted that although the difference in overall mood was significantly greater in the high-dose condition, the difference in scores is relatively small and we cannot determine whether the difference is *clinically* significant. In other words, we don't know if there were any *meaningful* differences for students in one condition versus another. The definition of clinically significant outcomes from animals is yet another important issue to explore. Beyond statistical differences, are there doses of HAI that result in more meaningful experiences and effects for humans? Differences between groups is an important finding but doesn't necessarily mean it was the HAI dose that impacted mood. Further analyses were conducted to test for associations between mood and HAI quantity.

Mood State and HAI Dose Correlations

Pearson *r* correlations were calculated between HAIS scores and mood at pretest and posttest. While there was no correlation between *pretest* mood and HAI, there was a significant correlation at *posttest*, $r\ (58) = 0.499$, $p < 0.001$. Table 3.1 provides the correlations, showing total HAI as well as human- and animal-initiated HAI. Mood is separated into the three dimensions of valence, calmness, and energetic arousal; total HAIS scores

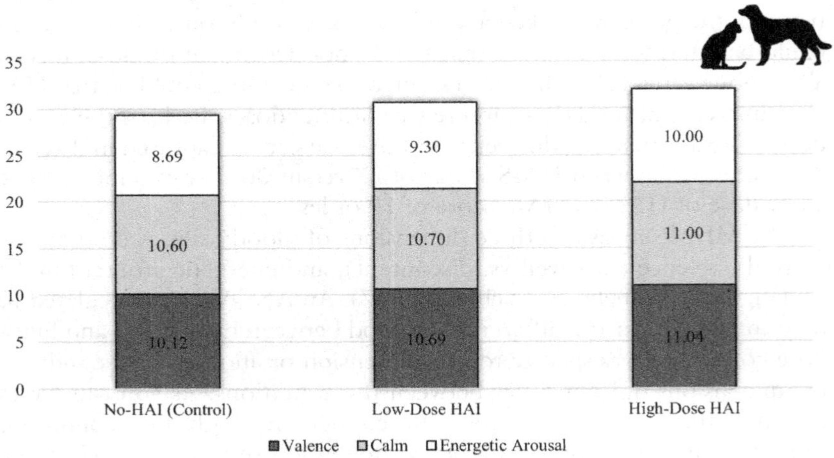

Fig. 3.2 Mood subscores across conditions. Graph showing mean scores for valence, calm, and energetic arousal across no-, low-, and high-dose HAI conditions. There were no significant differences in these mood dimensions

Table 3.1 Correlations between human–animal interaction and posttest mood

Human–animal interaction	*Valence*	*Calmness*	*Energetic arousal*
Human-initiated	0.487**	0.319*	0.352**
Animal-initiated	0.261*	0.385**	0.409**
Total HAI	0.429**	0.371**	0.402**

Note: The table provides correlations between HAI and three mood dimensions—valence, calm, and energetic arousal—in a laboratory study with 78 university students. Each of the dimensions was correlated with human-initiated, animal-initiated, and total HAI

**$p < 0.01$

*$p < 0.05$

correlated with all three dimensions. In addition, the strength of the correlation seems to differ by the source of the interaction, whether it was initiated by the human or the animal. Human-initiated interaction was most strongly correlated with mood valence while animal-initiated interaction was most strongly correlated with tension and energy level.

These findings could be interpreted to suggest that a human behaving toward an animal (e.g., petting a dog) impacts the human's emotion/affect while the animal behaving toward the human (e.g., dog sniffs and licks a client's hand) impacts the level of physical tension and energy. A search of the literature to date shows no studies addressing this question. Investigations of specific animal behaviors have focused on animal cognition as it relates to communication between dogs and humans (e.g., Polgárdi et al. 2000). More research is needed to confirm whether these are reliable findings. My hope in sharing it here is to provide an example of how dose can be defined and studied. Mean group differences and correlations are traditional ways to test outcomes within the social sciences. As was mentioned earlier, applying the medical model could provide a valuable perspective on AAI. Medicines are often tested in terms of dose–response relationships.

Dose–Response Relationships

In pharmacology, a medicine's ***dose–response relationship*** is the relationship between the amount of drug and the magnitude of the effect produced (Tallarida and Jacob 1979). White et al. (2013) discussed a dose–response relationship when studying the restorative effects of visiting nature. Using data from the Monitoring Engagement with the Natural Environment survey, they found participants reported greater restorative effects from some green spaces than others. They also found restoration correlated with visit duration; longer visits were associated with greater restorative feelings (e.g., calm, relaxed, refreshed).

With regard to psychological intervention, dose–effect research began with Howard et al. (1986) studying patient improvement in relation to the number of psychotherapy sessions attended. They found a significant correlation between these variables, which spurred further research. Several other studies found a positive correlation between number of sessions and improvement in well-being, symptoms, and functioning (Timulak 2008). Key among these studies is work by Kopta et al. (1994), who estimated a curvilinear relationship between number of sessions and recovery for patients with affective and anxiety disorders. Similarly, Warner et al. (2001) compared the treatment length–outcome relationship for patients in cognitive-behavioral versus psychodynamic psychotherapy. They found a dose–response relationship in both modalities, with differential treatment effects for varying perceptions of symptom severity. Given the dose–response relationship for other mental-health interventions, it stands to reason that AAI could be studied in a similar fashion. We could investigate a dose–response relationship between AAI process variables and outcomes. There may be many "active ingredients" in an AAI, and the literature suggests interacting with animals is one of them. In that context, I've examined the dose–response relationship between HAI and outcome variables, defining HAI dose as self-reported behavioral interaction and time spent with animals.

Dose–Response for Behavioral HAI

I calculated a *dose–response curve* using the same data described earlier, in which 75 students spent unstructured time with a dog or cat and reported on HAI and mood. A dose–response curve is a plot of the data where dose (i.e., HAI quantity) is treated as an independent variable plotted on the abscissa and the dependent variable (i.e., mood) plotted on the ordinate. In general, dose–response curves illustrate the relationship between the independent and dependent variables. Typically, increasing doses of the independent variable coincide with increasing levels of the dependent variable until reaching an upper bound where increasing dose has diminishing returns (Tallarida and Jacob 1979).

Figure 3.3 shows the dose–response curve for the relationship between HAI dose and mood. The *x*-axis shows doses of HAI (i.e., total HAIS scores) in 5-point increments from 0 to 60. The *y*-axis shows the percentage of students who showed an improvement in mood (valence and calm) from pre to post, with improvement defined as any increase in MDMS score from pretest to posttest. As you can see from the figure, the trend line for these data follows a hyperbolic curve, with response for valence and calm increasing sharply with increased dose from 0 to 15, then leveling off and even decreasing slightly with increased dose beyond 20. The trend line crosses the *y*-axis at 15 and 29 for valence and calm, respectively, while dose is 0. This represents participants in the control condition who experienced no HAI but reported improved mood at posttest. These data suggest the relationship between HAI and mood was not linear. In other

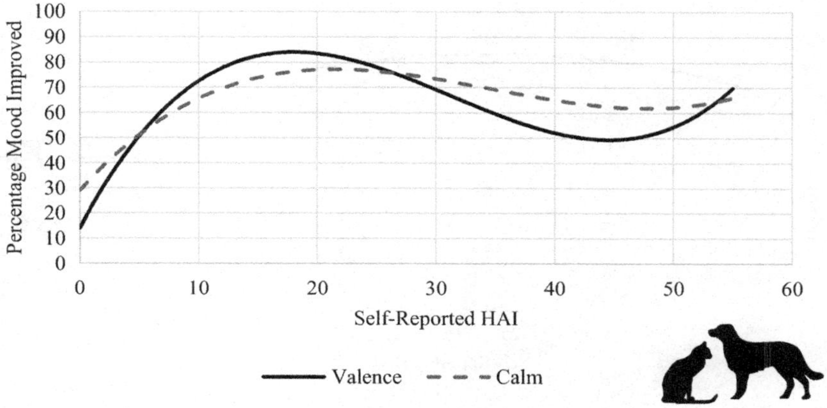

Fig. 3.3 Dose–response relationship for HAI and mood. Graph showing the relationship between HAI dose and reported mood in university students who spent unstructured time with a dog or cat. Dose was defined as HAIS score; response was defined as the percentage of participants reporting any improvement in mood from pretest to posttest

words, we cannot simply say "the more the merrier" for students in this study. Instead, it suggests that greater amounts of HAI were associated with improved mood, but only to a certain point. Increased HAI beyond a HAIS score of 20 did not result in proportionate improvements in mood. This kind of analysis could be important, when studied on a larger scale, in determining the ideal duration of individual sessions or amount of HAI needed for an encounter to have an impact.

Figure 3.4 is a dose–response curve showing the relationship between mood and HAI dose across several species. These data are from 50 college students who spent several minutes of unstructured interaction with a dog, a cat, or a rat. All interactions took place in the same laboratory observation room. As the figure shows, there was a similar dose–response relationship; as HAI quantity increased, the percentage of participants with a positive response increased. Again, the relationship appears to be curvilinear, with response increasing sharply at lower doses of HAI and then plateauing. In contrast to the previously discussed study, this investigation did not include a no-HAI control condition. No participants reported a dose of 0; the lowest dose of HAI reported with a dog, cat, or rat was a HAIS score of 4, 18, and 8 respectively.

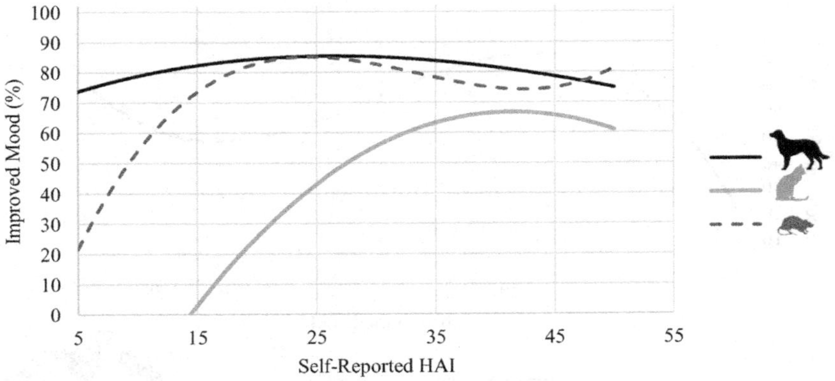

Fig. 3.4 Dose–response relationship for HAI and mood across species. Graph showing the relationship between HAI and mood. Dose–response curves are compared between college students who spent unstructured time with a dog, cat, or rat (n = 50). Response was strongest to the dog (n = 17), then the rat (n = 18), then the cat (n = 15)

This graph shows some differences in dose–response across species. Although the relationship between HAI and mood response appears to be hyperbolic in shape for those who interacted with a cat or rat, the line is relatively flat for those who interacted with a dog. In other words, response may not have been dependent on HAI dose when the animal was a dog. Whether participants reported lower or higher scores on the HAIS, there was a 75–88% response to interactions with a dog. In general, the response seemed to be the strongest for interaction with a dog, then rat, then cat. While the range of HAIS scores did not differ between the species, the percentage of participants with a response (i.e., mood improved from pre to post) did. Hyperbolic curves can be described in terms of an exponential-growth phase and a stationary phase. The data on cat and rat interactions have a similar pattern, but for the cat the exponential-growth phase starts at higher doses, has a more gradual slope, and the stationary phase occurs at a lower response. Taken together, these data suggest the student response to interacting with a rat was stronger than interacting with a cat. Follow-up research would be necessary to determine whether these dose–response curves represent the relationship between behavioral HAI and mood in the general population. In addition to comparing curves across different species, it may be useful to compare curves of individual animals within the same species (e.g., comparing two dogs or two cats). In equine-assisted psychotherapy, sessions often involve several horses in a pasture (Thomas and Lytle 2016). Over time, one could gather dose–response data on the individual horses of an equine-assisted psychotherapy and learning (EAP) practice to determine whether clients have different responses to different horses. These curves depict the dose–response relationship for the total HAIS score, representing an overall quantity of behavioral HAI. With a larger database, we could examine the dose–response relationship for individual behaviors or groups of behaviors.

Dose–response relationships can be explored across species, individual animals, and settings. These data show the dose–response curve when HAI dose is defined as scores on the HAIS. But HAI could be operationalized in many ways and detecting a reliable dose–response relationship will require detection of similar response patterns across various operational definitions. To that end, the following is a description of a study in which HAI dose was defined as time spent with animals rather than behavioral ratings.

Dose–Response for Time Spent

Each semester our university, like many institutions, holds a destress-with-pets event. These are events in which students can spend time with animals as a means of reducing the stress associated with mid-terms, finals, or any number of other sources of student stress. The programs are quite popular, and research suggests they have a positive impact on student well-being. According to Crossman and Kazdin (2015), over 900 colleges and universities in the U.S. utilize human–animal programming of some kind to help ameliorate student distress, ranging from therapeutic programs with specific treatment objectives to open campus activities wherein students spend unstructured time with an animal. Haggerty and Mueller (2017) studied the prevalence, structure, and policies of animal-assisted programming in colleges and universities. They surveyed 68 schools across the U.S. and found that 62% of them implemented some type of AAI for student stress.

On the more formal, therapeutic end, Binfet and Passmore (2016) studied an 8-week animal-assisted therapy (AAT) program aimed at reducing homesickness and increasing life satisfaction. Students who were randomly assigned to receive weekly group sessions with therapy dog/handler teams showed lower rates of homesickness and higher ratings of life satisfaction than students in a wait-list control group. Barker et al. (2017) investigated the effects of a college destress event on student perceptions of stressors and family support. Students spent 15 minutes with a therapy dog, then completed self-report measures. Saliva samples were collected, measuring physiological correlates of stress, before and after the intervention. Although physiological measures showed no differences in pre–post or treatment–control comparisons, self-reported stress was significantly different for both comparisons. The results suggest animal-assisted destress programming can positively impact students' perceived level of stress.

The destress-with-pets event on our campus is an animal-assisted activity (AAA). Dogs and cats from the community animal shelter come to campus for the afternoon. Each animal is in a cubicle with an animal handler (i.e., shelter staff or volunteer). Students can drop in and spend time with the animals anytime during the two-hour event. Student attendees can choose which animals they want to interact with and how much time they want to spend. The event is held during finals week each semester. For program evaluation, students attending the event are asked to complete a brief, anonymous survey. Next, I will share results form an analysis of this archival data, exploring HAI dose and response.

The archive includes 575 individuals attending the destress-with-pets event across four semesters. The participants were mostly students but could also have included faculty or staff, as the event is open to everyone on campus. Each semester, the event was held in the same room of the student union. The room is 11 m × 12 m, partitioned into nine 1.5 m × 2.5 m cubicles. Each cubicle would include one animal—a dog or cat—and an animal handler. The event is hosted and managed by the university's health-education office.

The program is evaluated with a student rating form, which is a 22 cm × 10 cm piece of paper, asking students to record the time of day and their stress level when entering and exiting the event. Stress was rated from 0 to 10, with 0 indicating "not at all stressed" and 10 indicating "completely stressed." Ratings for before and after the event were on either side of the rating form, so that at pretest, they only saw the questions about time of arrival and initial stress. The posttest side of the form asked about exit time and stress level, and included a space for written comments.

Student volunteers were seated at a table outside the entrance/exit to the event. As students approached the event, they were asked to complete the front side of the rating form. They were told to take it with them to the event and bring it back on their way out. When a student was done visiting the animals, they exited through the same door they entered; volunteers asked them to complete the back of the rating form. Completed forms were put into a lock box where they remained until they were entered into a spreadsheet after the event. With no names or identifying information on them, the student ratings were anonymous. This study involved analysis of the anonymous archival database from four semesters in 2016 and 2017. For the purposes of this analysis, HAI dose was defined as time spent with the animals at the event.

Participants spent up to 48 minutes at the event ($M = 13.80$, $SD = 9.14$), reporting variable stress levels upon arrival. Pretest stress ratings ranged from 0 to 10 ($M = 5.97$, $SD = 2.03$). Of the 575 participants in the sample, 90.2% ($n = 518$) reported a decrease in stress from pretest to posttest, 5.7% reported no change ($n = 33$), and 4.1% reported an increase in stress of 1 to 2 points ($n = 24$). Paired-samples t-tests showed reported stress decreased significantly from pretest ($M = 5.98$, $SD = 2.03$) to posttest ($M = 3.11$, $SD = 1.95$), $t\,(576) = 33.88$, $p < 0.001$. The change in stress ranged from a decrease of 10 points to an increase of 4 points ($M = -2.84$; $SD = 2.07$). A Pearson r correlation was calculated to determine whether change in stress was related to time spent at the event.

There was a weak, but significant correlation, $r\,(520) = -0.195$, $p < 0.001$. The data may have been affected by restricted range. As depicted in Fig. 3.5, although there were large ranges in time spent and stress reduction, most students spent between 3 and 20 minutes at the event (80%, $n = 424$) and reported a 1- to 5-point reduction in stress (71%, $n = 408$). To get a clearer picture of the relationship between time spent and stress reduction, I calculated a dose–response curve for these data, shown in Fig. 3.6. The x-axis represents HAI dose defined as time spent in minutes; the y-axis represents the percentage of participants who reported a positive response (i.e., reported stress decreased from pretest to posttest).

As the figure illustrates, responses were elicited at very low doses. The lowest dose recorded was 1 minute ($n = 4$), at which 75% of participants ($n = 3$) reported a response. The slope of the curve rises slightly between 1 minute (75% response, $n = 4$) and 15 minutes (88% response, $n = 358$) and then levels off. This slight curve indicates students responded at very low doses, increases in dose resulted in very slight increases in response, followed by a plateau at 90% response. Figure 3.6 shows the percentage of students responding at all. The dose–response curve in Fig. 3.7 shows the amount of stress reduction across minutes spent at the event. This curve

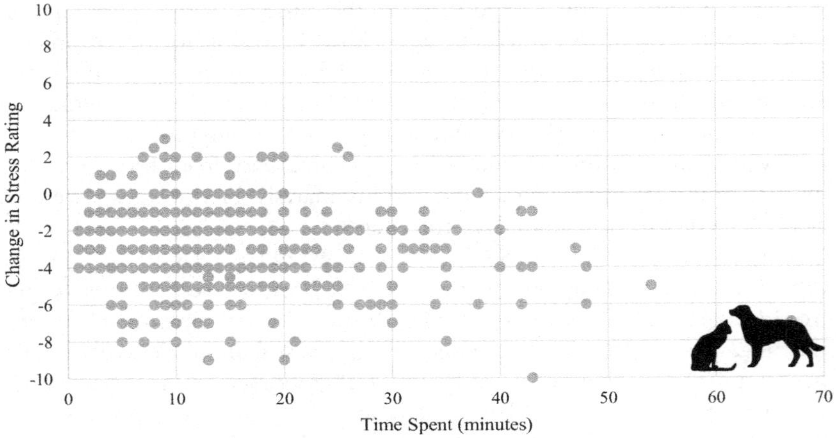

Fig. 3.5 Scatterplot of change in stress by time spent with animals. Data on the correlation between time spent at a university destress-with-pets event and reduced stress (n = 575). The graph shows the data were restricted in range for both time and stress

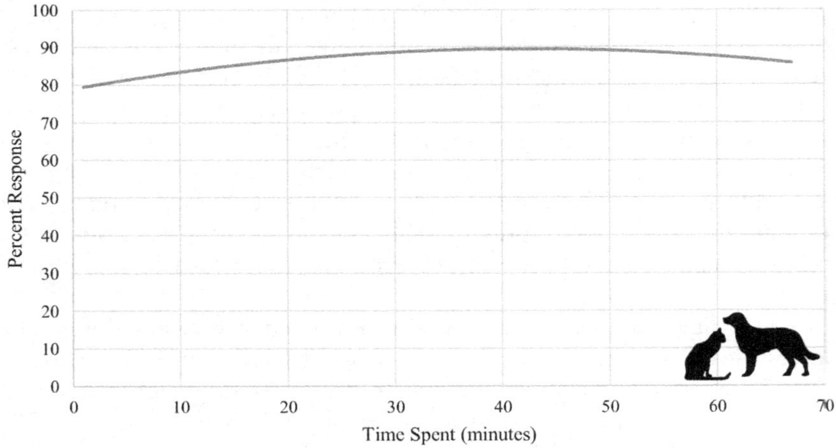

Fig. 3.6 Dose–response relationship for destress-with-pets. Depicts the dose–response curve for students attending a university destress-with-pets event. Dose was defined as time spent at the event, in minutes, and response was defined as the percentage of respondents who reported a decrease in stress from pretest to posttest

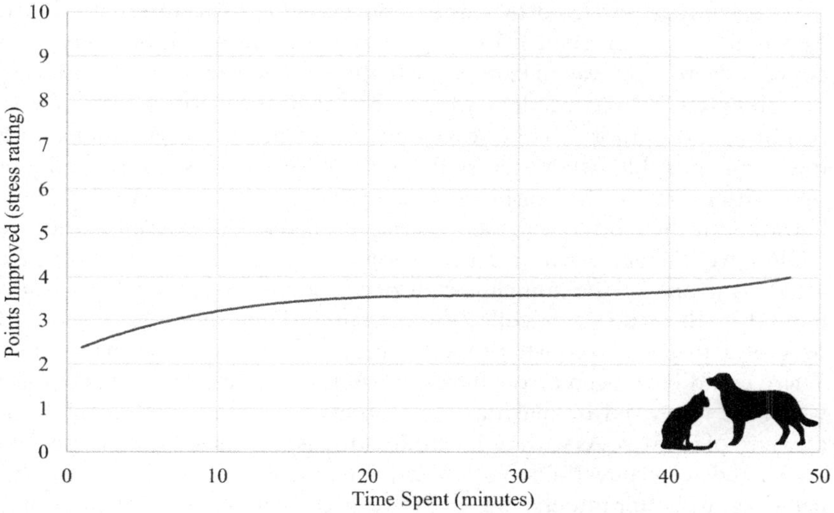

Fig. 3.7 Change in stress as a function of time spent with animals. Depicts the dose–response curve for destress-with-pets. Here, response is defined as the number of points improved on a stress-rating scale

illustrates increased improvement with greater time spent early on (i.e., 1–15 minutes), a leveling off until 35 minutes, and then a slight increase in improvement from 35 to 48 minutes.

From these data, we can see students overwhelmingly reported decreases in stress, and that stress level was correlated with length of time spent visiting with animals. The dose–response curves indicate that response tended to happen at low doses for most people, with diminishing returns after 15 minutes. Similarly, increased dose was associated with increased benefit, but just to approximately 15 minutes. Taken together, these data suggest that when dose was defined by time spent, students could benefit from low doses (i.e., just a few minutes of interaction with animals), important information when developing university destress programs. This is consistent with the study by Barker et al. in which students spent 15 minutes with a therapy dog. Similarly, Crossman et al. (2015) found reductions in depressed mood and anxiety for students spending 7–10 minutes with an animal.

This study is restricted by some important threats to internal validity. Although it is assumed that time spent at the event was time spent with animals, there is no way of knowing whether that is true. Interactions were not observed and recorded, so we don't know if they visited with animals or not. Because more than one student could be visiting an animal at a time, it is possible other factors helped reduce stress, such as spending time with other students or just taking a break from classes. We also don't know about the kinds of interactions that occurred. For example, students could have interacted with a cat or a dog or both. They could have interacted with one of the animals or all of the animals. The analysis is also limited by the crude data collection measures. Time spent was calculated by subtracting their reported time of entrance from the time they exited. There could have been errors in recording these times. This investigation would be improved by making direct observations and using a validated measure of distress. As with other studies discussed in this book, these data are shared to inspire thinking and inquiry into AAI. Could you use this paradigm to better understand AAI in your clinical practice or laboratory?

Summary and Conclusion on HAI Dose

This chapter has explored the concept of dose, a term rarely used in the AAI literature. When discussed, researchers describe dose of the intervention as a whole, defined as number of intervention sessions, duration of the sessions, or length of treatment overall. This is consistent with dose–response research on traditional office-based psychotherapy (Howard et al. 1986; Timulak 2008). However, studying specific components of an intervention can allow for greater understanding of an intervention's efficacy. Including an animal in an intervention adds a layer of complexity. Claims that an AAI is effective, and that animals in general are good for human health and well-being, must be borne out through research examining the animal component of the intervention. Variables such as session frequency and duration or length of treatment cannot provide evidence for or against the animal's role in positive intervention outcomes. Following up on the call for HAI analysis in Chap. 2, research was described examining the dose–response relationship between HAI and distress reduction.

Two studies were described—one basic and one applied—examining HAI dose. In the laboratory, dose was experimentally manipulated to compare low-dose HAI, high-dose HAI, and no-HAI control conditions. Students randomly assigned to experience a high dose of HAI, defined by

HAIS scores, showed greater distress reduction than those in the no-HAI control condition. Although the data were trending such that low-dose HAI was associated with lower levels of distress reduction than high-dose HAI, the difference was not significant. More research is necessary to determine whether there are critical doses. Are there quantities of HAI that tip the scales for improved well-being? Or is HAI an all-or-none variable as it has been studied thus far? Research on time spent with animals suggests positive effects of HAI occur relatively quickly, within a few minutes. In the laboratory, we found no difference in mood whether students spent 2 or 4 minutes with an animal. In the applied setting, where students could drop in to spend as much time as they liked with animals, most responded within 15 minutes.

Dose–response relationships for both studies followed a similar curve. Positive responses (i.e., improved mood, decreased stress) occurred at low doses, accelerated rapidly, then leveled off. This was true whether dose was defined as quantity of behavioral HAI measured with the HAIS or time spent at an animal-related event. The dose–response curves suggest the relationship was curvilinear. Future studies should expand investigations to other animals and a variety of dose operationalizations.

Taken together, the research described here suggests humans may experience distress reduction or improved mood at relatively low doses of HAI. After a short visit with animals, students reported feeling less stressed, more calm, and happier. Increased HAI provides some increased benefit, but only to a certain point. This is important for intervention efficiency, for the sake of the clients and animals. For instance, if a client can benefit from 15 minutes visiting with an animal, there is no need to conduct 30-minute visits. Shorter sessions could mean less burden on therapy animals, an important aspect of therapy animal welfare (Enders-Slegers et al. 2019). More laboratory-based research is necessary to disentangle the role of HAI dose in AAI outcomes. The research described here warrants replication with larger, more diverse samples of humans and animals.

For AAI practitioners, calculating dose–response curves for your practice, for specific therapy animals, or for your individual clients could be useful. Just as with medications, optimal dose may be specific to the individual client, based on biological and psychological factors and situational context. The research described here measured the association between HAI and stress, mood, and anxiety. These variables fall into the broader category of psychological distress, a common variable studied in AAI outcome research. Our research team has been studying this broader outcome—a decrease in distress or a lift in mood. We call this reduction in psychological distress an anodyne effect, discussed next in Chap. 4.

References

Barker, S. B., Barker, R. T., McCain, N. L., & Schubert, C. M. (2017). The effect of a canine-assisted activity on college student perceptions of family supports and current stressors. *Anthrozoös, 30*(4), 595–606.

Binfet, J. T., & Passmore, H. A. (2016). Hounds and homesickness: The effects of an animal-assisted therapeutic intervention for first-year university students. *Anthrozoös, 29*(3), 441–454.

Cracknell, D., White, M. P., Pahl, S., Nichols, W. J., & Depledge, M. H. (2016). Marine biota and psychological well-being: A preliminary examination of dose–response effects in an aquarium setting. *Environment and Behavior, 48*(10), 1242–1269.

Crossman, M. K. (2017). Effects of interactions with animals on human psychological distress. *Journal of Clinical Psychology, 73*(7), 761–784.

Crossman, M. K., & Kazdin, A. E. (2015). Animal visitation programs in colleges and universities: An efficient model for reducing student stress. In A. H. Fine (Ed.), *Handbook on animal-assisted therapy* (pp. 333–337). Academic Press.

Crossman, M. K., Kazdin, A. E., & Knudson, K. (2015). Brief unstructured interaction with a dog reduces distress. *Anthrozoös, 28*(4), 649–659.

Dallimer, M., Irvine, K. N., Skinner, A. M., Davies, Z. G., Rouquette, J. R., Maltby, L. L., et al. (2012). Biodiversity and the feel-good factor: Understanding associations between self-reported human well-being and species richness. *Bioscience, 62*(1), 47–55.

Enders-Slegers, M. J., Hediger, K., Beetz, A., Jegatheesan, B., & Turner, D. (2019). Animal-assisted intervention within an international perspective: Trends, research, and practices. In A. H. Fine (Ed.), *Handbook on animal-assisted therapy: Foundations and guidelines for animal-assisted interventions* (5th ed., pp. 465–478). San Diego, CA: Elsevier.

Esposito, L., McCune, S., Griffin, J. A., & Maholmes, V. (2011). Directions in human–animal interaction research: Child development, health, and therapeutic interventions. *Child Development Perspectives, 5*(3), 205–211.

Fournier, A. K., Berry, T. D., Letson, E. E., & Chanen, R. (2016). The human-animal interaction scale: Development and evaluation. *Anthrozoös, 29*(3), 455–467.

Fuller, R. A., Irvine, K. N., Devine-Wright, P., Warren, P. H., & Gaston, K. J. (2007). Psychological benefits of greenspace increase with biodiversity. *Biology Letters, 3*(4), 390–394.

Haggerty, J. M., & Mueller, M. K. (2017). Animal-assisted stress reduction programs in higher education. *Innovative Higher Education, 42*(5–6), 379–389.

Howard, K. I., Kopta, S. M., Krause, M. S., & Orlinsky, D. E. (1986). The dose–effect relationship in psychotherapy. *American Psychologist, 41*(2), 159.

Jones, M. G., Rice, S. M., & Cotton, S. M. (2019). Incorporating animal-assisted therapy in mental health treatments for adolescents: A systematic review of canine assisted psychotherapy. *PLoS One, 14*(1), e0210761.

Kamioka, H., Okada, S., Tsutani, K., Park, H., Okuizumi, H., Handa, S., et al. (2014). Effectiveness of animal-assisted therapy: A systematic review of randomized controlled trials. *Complementary Therapies in Medicine, 22*(2), 371–390.

Kopta, S. M., Howard, K. I., Lowry, J. L., & Beutler, L. E. (1994). Patterns of symptomatic recovery in psychotherapy. *Journal of Consulting and Clinical Psychology, 62*(5), 1009.

Merriam-Webster. (2019). Dose. Retrieved from https://www.merriam-webster.com/dictionary/dose?utm_campaign=sd&utm_medium=serp&utm_source=jsonld.

Nimer, J., & Lundahl, B. (2007). Animal-assisted therapy: A meta-analysis. *Anthrozoös, 20*(3), 225–238.

Polgárdi, R., Topál, J., & Csányi, V. (2000). Intentional behaviour in dog-human communication: An experimental analysis of "showing" behaviour in the dog. *Animal Cognition, 3*(3), 159–166.

Serpell, J., McCune, S., Gee, N., & Griffin, J. A. (2017). Current challenges to research on animal-assisted interventions. *Applied Developmental Science, 21*(3), 223–233.

Tallarida, R. J., & Jacob, L. S. (1979). *The dose—Response relation in pharmacology*. New York, NY: Springer.

Thomas, L., & Lytle, M. (2016). *Transforming therapy through horses: Case stories teaching the Eagala model in action*. Santaquin, UT: Eagala.

Timulak, L. (2008). *Research in psychotherapy and counseling*. Thousand Oaks, CA: Sage.

Vitztum, C. (2013). Human–animal interaction: A concept analysis. *International Journal of Nursing Knowledge, 24*(1), 30–36.

Warner, L. K., Herron, W. G., Javier, R. A., Patalano, F., Sisenwein, F., & Primavera, L. H. (2001). A comparison of dose–response curves in cognitive–behavioral and psychodynamic psychotherapies. *Journal of Clinical Psychology, 57*(1), 63–73.

White, M. P., Pahl, S., Ashbullby, K., Herbert, S., & Depledge, M. H. (2013). Feelings of restoration from recent nature visits. *Journal of Environmental Psychology, 35*, 40–51.

Wilhelm, P., & Schoebi, D. (2007). Assessing mood in daily life structural validity, sensitivity to change, and reliability of a short scale to measure three basic dimensions of mood. *European Journal of Psychological Assessment, 23*(4), 258–267. https://doi.org/10.1027/1015-5759.23.4.258.

Wilkie, K. D., Germain, S., & Theule, J. (2016). Evaluating the efficacy of equine therapy among at-risk youth: A meta-analysis. *Anthrozoös, 29*(3), 377–393.

CHAPTER 4

Animals as Anodyne

Abstract An anodyne is something that soothes, calms, or comforts. In this chapter, I argue that animals facilitate intervention, in part, by acting as an anodyne—eliciting a superficial, perhaps temporary, reduction in distress (i.e., improved mood, reduced tension or anxiety). Just as an aspirin can relieve the pain of a headache superficially, without necessarily treating the underlying cause, interacting with an animal may result in a reduction of subjective distress, without necessarily treating the underlying source of the distress. This lift in mood may be an end in and of itself or may help to facilitate a therapy or learning process aimed at longer-term change. Various research on animal-assisted intervention (AAI) implies an anodyne effect, wherein interactions with animals are associated with reduced physical or emotional distress. This chapter reviews a sample of those studies in the context of an anodyne effect and describes experimental research testing animals as anodyne.

Keywords Anodyne • Animal-assisted intervention • Distress reduction • Human–animal interaction

The impact of animal-assisted intervention (AAI) on human health and well-being is a burgeoning research topic. Studies in this area regularly conclude with statements regarding the need for a theory or framework from which to study AAI. I review outcomes measured to date and

A. K. Fournier, *Animal-Assisted Intervention*,
https://doi.org/10.1007/978-3-030-32972-3_4

introduce a superordinate construct which encompasses many of these outcomes. The construct provides a framework for interpreting previous findings and developing testable research questions regarding a potential role of animals in assisting or facilitating intervention—animals elicit an anodyne effect.

Anodyne Effect

An anodyne is defined as something that soothes, calms, or comforts (Merriam-Webster 2019). I suggest that one important way an animal may impact human health and well-being is by acting as an anodyne—causing a superficial, perhaps temporary, lift in mood state or subjective well-being. More specifically, I propose that engaging with animals causes humans to feel happier, calmer, and/or less stressed or distressed. Just as an aspirin can relieve the pain of a headache without treating the underlying cause (e.g., muscle tension, vascular issues), an anodyne effect from human–animal interaction (HAI) alone can impact subjective distress, but may not necessarily treat the underlying source of the distress. Although not labeled as such, various research on AAI implies an anodyne effect, wherein interactions with animals are associated with reduced physical or emotional distress. We can see examples of this effect within animal-assisted therapies and activities.

Anodyne in Animal-Assisted Therapies

Animal-assisted therapies (AAT) are interventions that incorporate animals in achieving a variety of health-related goals or objectives (American Veterinary Medical Association 2019). These therapies can address physical and/or psychological pain, distress, or functioning. The literature provides several examples of AAT wherein the measured outcome could be conceptualized as an anodyne effect.

Psychotherapy and Counseling

Practitioners describe the use of animals in psychotherapy or counseling as having many benefits, including those that could fit under the broader umbrella of an anodyne effect. For example, Chandler suggests watching animals could at the very least elicit a smile and could have the important effect of calming and soothing (2017). Fine (2019a) shared observations from practice, describing animals putting clients at ease and regulating the emotional climate of the therapy session as part of rapport building. Beyond these clinical descriptions, empirical research suggests improved mood and reduced stress are consistent outcomes.

Kern-Godal et al. (2016) conducted a phenomenological investigation of equine-assisted therapy, in which the patient–horse relationship was identified by participants with substance-use disorders. Emotional affect was a key factor identified within the patient–horse relationship; participants indicated their relationship with the horse resulted in feeling happy, calm, and safe.

In a study of animal-assisted psychotherapy for residential adolescents, Muela et al. (2017) found that residents in an AAT treatment group had improvements in depressed mood compared to the control group.

Bivens et al. (2007) conducted an open clinical trial on the effects of equine-assisted experiential therapy in a residential group setting. Self-report data indicated significant improvements in psychological distress at posttreatment and six months follow-up. Hoffmann et al. (2009) investigated the effect of therapy dogs on the treatment of hospitalized patients with acute depression. Compared with a nonanimal control condition, patients in the animal-assisted condition reported reduced state anxiety. It was suggested that the reduced anxiety could enhance psychotherapeutic strategies and improve motivation. Berget et al. (2011) conducted a randomized controlled trial (RCT) testing the effects of an AAT with farm animals for psychiatric patients. After the 12-week intervention, participants showed reductions in anxiety and depression. Most notably, anxiety was reduced in the treatment group but not in the control group, while depression was reduced at follow-up for both groups.

Physical, Occupational, or Recreational Therapies

Although there is a greater focus in the literature on AAI for mental health, animals are also used in interventions targeting physical health and functioning. Wood et al. (2017) conducted a systematic review of the occupational therapy literature on AAT for institutionalized individuals with dementia. They found ten studies meeting their criteria and mapped them onto the lived-environment-life-quality model. All of the studies involved one or more dogs and a health practitioner (e.g., physical therapist, occupational therapist, therapeutic recreation specialist). Outcomes were mapped onto three quality-of-life domains—ability to function, engagement, and well-being. Each of the studies found outcomes related to the well-being domain. Improved affect or decreased depression was indicated in five of the studies and reduced agitation or irritability was indicated in four of the studies.

As an example of an individual study on AAT for physical treatments, Kreivinienė and Perttula (2014) conducted qualitative research on AAT using dolphins. These authors actually referred to dolphins acting as anodyne. Researchers interviewed ten families raising children with cerebral palsy who participated in a dolphin-assisted therapy program. Family members described the dolphins as helping to calm the children, much like a prescription drug would.

Anodyne in Animal-Assisted Activities

As mentioned earlier, animal-assisted activities (AAAs) are nontreatment interventions in which animals are incorporated into activities to promote human health and well-being (American Veterinary Medical Association 2019). Examples include brief animal visits and organized activities with animals. These activities are often provided in hospitals, nursing homes, and school settings.

Hospitals and Medical Centers

A significant number of hospitals and medical centers provide animal visits to their patients, family members, and medical staff. Murthy et al. (2015) surveyed members of the Society for Healthcare Epidemiology of America. When asked if AAA was allowed in their facility, 82% said yes. Of the hospitals located in the U.S., 89% allowed AAA. Bringing animals into healthcare settings has some unique challenges and opportunities. For a more thorough review and suggestions on AAA in healthcare settings, see Barker and Barker (2019). Regarding an anodyne effect, research has demonstrated AAA programs in medical settings are associated with reduced anxiety and fear, as well as increased positive affect.

Dogs on Call is one such program in which therapy dogs and their handlers visit patients in medical settings. The program has been studied extensively and shows several positive outcomes. Regarding an anodyne effect, research suggests the dog visits help to reduce anxiety, fear, and stress. In a study on anxiety and pain in hospitalized children, participants who received dog visits reported lower anxiety at posttest (Barker et al.

2015). In another study, hospitalized psychiatric patients participated in a group activity with a therapy dog or traditional recreational therapy. Anxiety was significantly lower after the animal-related activity; this was true for patients with a variety of diagnoses (Barker and Dawson 1998). Barker and colleagues also studied the effects of dog visits on fear and anxiety in psychiatric patients before receiving electroconvulsive therapy. Results showed significant reductions in fear and anxiety for patients receiving the dog visits (Barker et al. 2003).

Nursing Homes

Holcomb et al. (1997) studied the effects of an aviary on men in an adult day care facility. This single-case reversal design indicated the presence of the aviary was associated with reduced depression. A study by Oliva et al. (2010) examined the effects of weekly dog visits for elderly residents of a nursing home. Residents were encouraged to spend time with, pet, walk, and groom therapy dogs. Facility staff reported improved mood (i.e., reduced irritability, increased happiness) among other outcomes.

Schools

Animals are present in a variety of school settings, from preschools to universities. Many studies in school settings address the impact of animals on learning and cognitive abilities. Here, I provide some examples where an anodyne effect was among the outcomes. Beetz (2013) studied the effects of a dog in the classroom for third graders. The dog was present in a classroom one day per week, compared with a control classroom. Students reported increased positive emotion in class and a more positive attitude toward school; both were suggested as important precursors to effective learning. Regarding higher education, many colleges and universities implement AAA programs to help students with anxiety and depression or stress in general. For example, Stewart et al. (2014) studied the effects of an animal-assisted outreach program on college-student anxiety and loneliness. Students reported significant decreases in both variables following the intervention. In a similar study, Grajfoner et al. (2017) studied a brief AAA in which university students spent unstructured time with dogs. The data showed improvement in self-reported mood, anxiety, and well-being. These effects were strongest when interactions occurred without the animal handler, eliminating the possibility that outcomes resulted from human social interaction.

As you can see, there are many examples of AAI being associated with reduced negative emotions like anxiety, fear, stress, and irritability and increased positive emotions such as happiness, calm, and relaxation. The literature reviewed here is just a sample of the research on this topic. Researchers interested in the impact of animals on human health and well-being have also conducted research on HAI outside of any formal intervention context. Similarly, these HAI studies measure constructs that could be considered evidence of an anodyne effect.

Anodyne in Human–Animal Interaction Research

Turner reviewed literature on human–cat interactions across a span of 30 years (2017). Regarding the benefits of cats, research suggests participants experience improvements in mood following interactions with pet cats. In a laboratory experiment, Aydin et al. (2012) found the presence of an unfamiliar dog resulted in less psychological distress and a greater sense of well-being for participants who had been socially excluded. Among other psychosocial variables, the researchers found that participants' positive emotions were higher in the presence of a dog, compared to participants in a no-dog condition. They suggest dogs serve as stand-ins for humans, mediating social isolation.

Beyond these individual examples, the more summative literature also indicates a relationship between HAI and anodyne-like effects. Crossman (2017) synthesized the research literature on HAI regarding distress reduction as an outcome. The review examined psychological distress following the definition by Drapeau et al. (2012), which includes the experience of mood and anxiety resulting in emotional hardship and potential associated physiological symptoms. The author concludes animals can benefit via distress reduction and calls for more in-depth examination of HAI as a phenomenon, beyond AAT outcome studies.

The studies reviewed here indicate that among the many outcomes measured when investigating AAI, improvements in emotion or mood, including decreased distress, are common outcomes. My research team and I have studied this, referring to it as an anodyne effect, in both applied and basic research, examining the relationship between anodyne-related outcomes and behavioral HAI. Here I discuss two studies designed to investigate an anodyne effect—a correlational study from an AAT client archive and a laboratory experiment with university students.

Human–Horse Interaction and Anodyne

Our research team is fortunate to collaborate with a local provider of equine-assisted psychotherapy and learning (EAP). It has become common practice for clients to complete a Human–Animal Interaction Scale (HAIS) (Fournier et al. 2016) and distress rating for each session. This is used to track both clients and therapy animals over time. This practice has been helpful to identify changes in HAI between the clients and horses and to tie client outcomes to interactions with the horses. At intake, clients at the center have the opportunity to contribute their data to a de-identified database for archival research. Participating in the research is voluntary and is not connected to access to treatment or the nature of treatment. The archival data contain scores on the HAIS, distress ratings, and comments about the session. The archive does not include any identifiable information nor any information on diagnostic status, treatment plans, or treatment progress.

A study was conducted to assess the relationship between human–horse interaction, subjective distress, and psychosocial learning. The study is described in greater detail elsewhere (Fournier et al. 2018). Here, I focus on distress ratings in the context of an anodyne effect. Participants were 112 men and women who attended one or more EAP sessions; data are from one individual or group session for each client. Materials included the HAIS and the Subjective Units of Distress Scale (SUDS), a Likert scale on which an individual rates their distress from 0 to 10 (Wolpe 1990). The SUDS is established as a valid measure of distress and can be used to determine progress in therapy (e.g., Kaplan et al. 1995; Rothbaum et al. 2005). In this study, participants rated current mood and anxiety, each on a 0–10 scale, where 0 indicated "none" and 10 indicated "worst ever." Clients completed a SUDS for before the session and after the session (i.e., pretest–posttest). They also completed a HAIS form, reporting their behavioral interactions with the horses.

Paired-samples *t*-tests on SUDS ratings showed decreases in anxiety from pretest ($M = 3.57$, $SD = 2.73$) to posttest ($M = 2.03$, $SD = 2.64$), $t(90) = 5.26$, $p < 0.001$ and improvements in mood from pretest ($M = 3.77$, $SD = 2.24$) to posttest ($M = 2.24$, $SD = 2.40$), $t(83) = 6.19$, $p < 0.001$. Table 4.1 shows correlations between HAI and SUDS ratings at pretest and posttest. The data support an anodyne effect; HAI was correlated with posttest ratings but not pretest ratings for both mood and anxiety. Furthermore, human-initiated HAI seemed to be more strongly associated with reduced distress than animal-initiated HAI.

Table 4.1 Correlations between HAI and distress in equine-assisted psychotherapy and learning

	Mood		*Anxiety*	
	Pre	*Post*	*Pre*	*Post*
Human-initiated	−0.152	**−0.344****	−0.096	**−0.393****
Animal-initiated	−0.175	**−0.263***	−0.034	−0.196
Total HAI	−0.161	**−0.322***	−0.070	**−0.356****

Note: The table provides coefficients for correlations between HAI and subjective distress ratings (i.e., mood, anxiety) before and after an EAP session. HAI was correlated with distress at posttest but not pretest. Significant correlations are in bold

**$p < 0.001$
*$p < 0.05$

Connecting this to the dose question in Chap. 3, Fig. 4.1 shows the dose–response curve for these data. Note that both mood and anxiety follow a similar pattern, although the overall response for mood was greater than the response for anxiety. The curve is less hyperbolic and more flat, with most doses resulting in a response rate between 60% and 80%. The growth phase prior to plateau is very gradual. Looking back at Fig. 3.4 in Chap. 3, these curves resemble the response curve for participants who interacted with dogs and are quite different from that of participants who interacted with a cat or rat.

Overall, these data provide support for an anodyne effect, with increasing HAI dose associated with a greater anodyne effect. This applied research was correlational and thus limited to conclusions about *associations* rather than evidence of HAI *causing* or *eliciting* an anodyne effect. We followed up this study with an experiment to test for causal evidence. Given the similarities between dose–response curves for HAI with dogs and horses, and the fact that these animals are often used in AAI (Fine 2019b), we compared HAI with both a horse and a dog to a control condition to explore similarities and differences between the species in an anodyne effect.

Anodyne Across Species

A laboratory study[1] was conducted to test for an anodyne effect. University students participated in a group AAI session randomly assigned to include tan experiential learning session designed to facilitate learning about

[1] For a more thorough description of the study, see Fournier et al., in press).

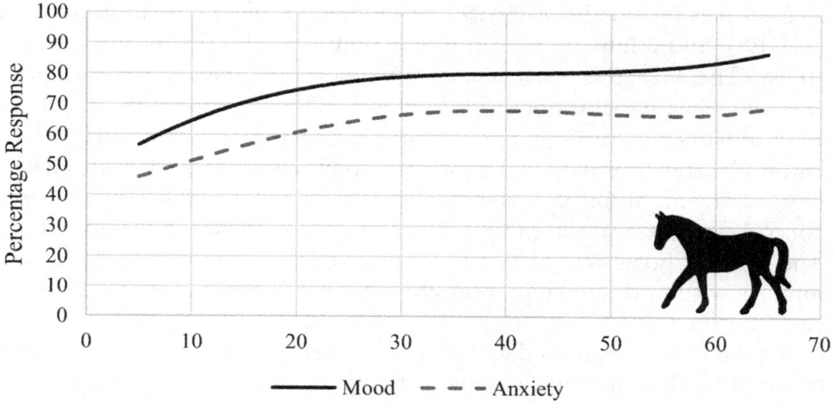

Fig. 4.1 Dose–response in equine-assisted psychotherapy and learning. Depicts dose–response curve for subjective distress ratings and percentage of clients reporting less distress from pre- to post-session (n = 112)

problem-solving, self when problem-solving, and self in group tasks. We predicted sessions involving animals would result in higher positive emotion and lower negative emotion scores than control sessions. Since research comparing horses and dogs is sparse and inadequate to support a priori interspecies predictions, comparisons between dog and horse conditions were exploratory.

We held a total of 12 group sessions (5 horse, 3 dog, 4 control), each taking place in the same enclosed horse arena. The arena was supplied with props for experiential learning (e.g., cones, barrels, blocks, toys). Participants were 45 undergraduate students in psychology. Consistent with the general population of students in the psychology department, the sample was largely White[2] (84%) women (80%) of traditional college age (M = 20.45, SD = 3.58). The animals were therapy animals that lived at the EAP center and had been involved in EAP for four years before the study began. The horse was a 30-year-old gelding Paint who served in Eagala-model EAP services. The dog was a 9-year-old neutered Labrador Retriever who had completed Canine Good Citizen and Therapy Dog International training.

[2] 6.7% identified as Native American (n = 3), 4.4% identified as African American or Black (n = 2), and 2.2% identified as Asian (n = 1).

Materials included the HAIS, the modified differential emotions scale (MDES), and a human–human interaction scale (HHIS) created for the study.[3] The MDES is a self-report instrument designed to measure positive and negative emotions (Fredrickson 2004; Galanakis et al. 2016). Respondents rate the degree to which they experience each of 20 different emotions—ten positive (e.g., joyful, happy, amused) and ten negative (e.g., irritated, suspicious, annoyed). The inanimate object used in the control condition was a 1 m × 1.3 m tan decommissioned rocking horse. The rocking horse served as a control, providing a four-legged being to interact with and allowing researchers to use the same instructions for each session.

Similar to university studies described earlier, participants were recruited through in-class announcements, offering extra credit for participation. To reduce selection bias, the study was described as "a study on group experiential learning" and did not mention animals. Sign-ups were posted by session and were scheduled on the same day and time, across several weeks during the 2017–2018 and 2018–2019 academic years. Cluster random assignment (Bloom et al. 1999) was implemented where each session was randomly assigned to one of the three conditions (i.e., horse, dog, or control).

Students were transported to and from the ranch by researchers. All sessions followed the Equine-Assisted Growth and Learning Association (Eagala) model (Eagala 2019) and were co-facilitated by the same licensed mental-health specialist and animal specialist. Facilitators, both certified in equine- and canine-assisted therapy, instructed participants to complete a task that involved (1) using and labeling props to (2) create a path toward a goal, and then (3) bringing the four-legged being (i.e., horse, dog, or rocking horse) through the path to the goal. Engaging with an inanimate object in the control condition avoided some important cofounds, as AAI can differ from traditional intervention beyond the mere presence of an animal (e.g., novelty, experiential modality, setting, provider). These variables were held constant in the present study to bet-

[3] The HHIS was created to identify any differences in social interaction among participants across the three conditions. This is a 19-item rating scale similar in form to the HAIS. After observing a session, researchers rated, from 0, indicating "not at all," to 4, indicating "a great deal," the extent to which they observed various interactive behaviors between group members. Reliability analysis, via Cronbach's alpha, suggests the instrument had adequate internal consistency ($\alpha = 0.73$).

ter attribute any anodyne effect to the animal rather than other variables. During the task, researchers unobtrusively observed and recorded behavior on the HAIS. Once the task was completed, participants processed the session with the facilitators and completed the HAIS and MDES. Then researchers gave students their extra credit, debriefed them, and brought them back to campus.

HAIS scores were compared between horse and dog sessions. Total HAI was higher in the dog condition ($M = 31.78$, $SD = 7.27$) than in the horse condition ($M = 22.46$, $SD = 4.14$), $t(6) = -2.37$, $p = 0.05$. Figure 4.2 shows mean ratings for individual behaviors, separated by species, showing which behaviors were similar and different. While quite a few items were

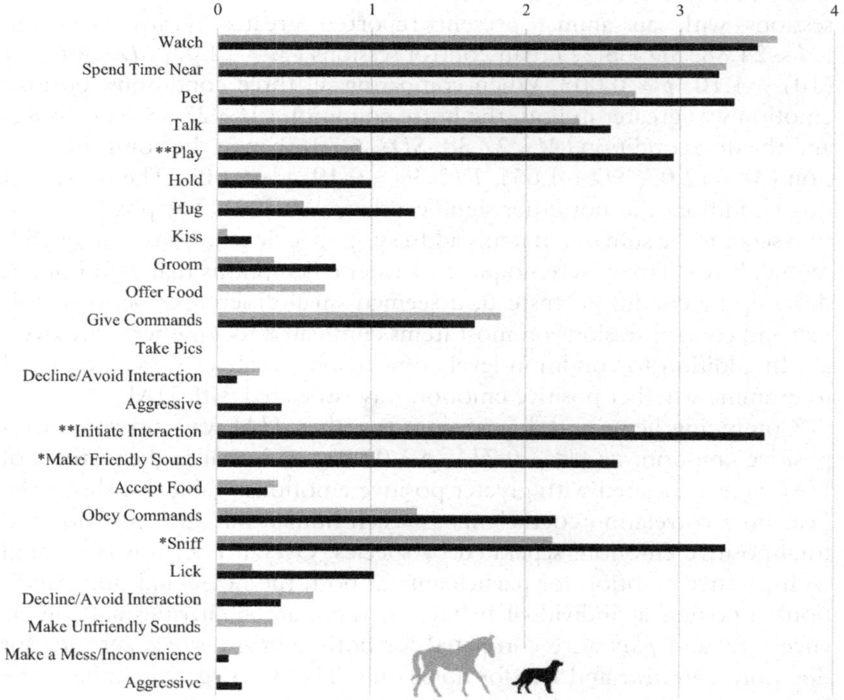

Fig. 4.2 Behavioral HAI with horse versus dog. Graph shows mean HAIS ratings for university students in a group-experiential learning session that included a horse, a dog, or a plush rocking horse. $^{**}p < 0.001$, $^{*}p < 0.05$

rated higher in the dog condition, the items that were *significantly* different were *play*, *initiate interaction*, *make friendly sounds*, and *sniff*. Note that *play* is the only human-initiated behavior and the rest of the differences were for animal-initiated behaviors. Participants perceived the dog to be more interactive than the horse.

The anodyne effect was tested by comparing positive and negative emotion between sessions with animals and the control condition. Negative emotion did not differ by condition, but negative emotions were rated relatively low. There may have been a floor effect, wherein baseline scores were so low there was no room for reduction in negative emotion. Since this was a nonclinical sample of college students, it makes sense that they would report low levels for negative emotions (e.g., sad, guilty, angry). However, there was a difference for positive emotion; students in sessions with an animal present reported greater positive emotion ($M = 24.88$, $SD = 5.27$) than control sessions ($M = 12.07$, $SD = 4.65$), $t\ (10) = 4.10$, $p = 0.002$. When comparing all three conditions, positive emotion was greater in both the horse condition ($M = 23.38$, $SD = 4.32$) and the dog condition ($M = 27.38$, $SD = 6.70$) than in the control condition ($M = 12.07$, $SD = 4.65$), $F\ (2, 9) = 9.19$, $p = 0.007$. The horse and dog conditions did not differ significantly ($p = 0.305$). The positive emotion score is the sum of ten items addressing specific emotions (e.g., joyful, serene, love). There were no particular items/emotions that stood out as differing by condition. Instead, it seemed small differences between animal and control sessions on most items cumulated to a higher score overall. In addition to condition-level comparisons, analyses were conducted to examine whether positive emotion was associated with HAI.

Combining horse and dog sessions together, HAI was correlated with positive emotion, $r\ (41) = 0.711$, $p < 0.001$, such that higher ratings of HAI were associated with greater positive emotions. Table 4.2 shows the Pearson r correlation coefficients for each human-initiated behavior and total positive emotion, separated by species. Overall HAI was correlated with positive emotion for participants in both the horse and dog conditions. Looking at individual behaviors, there are similarities and differences. *Pet* and *play* were correlated for both animals, *watch* and *hug* for dog only, and *near* and *talk* for horse only. The two negative, undesirable behaviors (*decline/avoid interaction*, *aggressive behavior*) were rated very low and not related to emotion. Neither were *kiss*, *groom*, *offer food*, *give commands*, and *take pics*. Thinking about the individual behaviors that do and do not correlate, I wonder if there is an underlying factor. For example, *grooming*, *offering food*, and *giving commands* to an animal are all fairly

Table 4.2 Correlation of human-initiated HAI and positive emotion, by species

Behavior	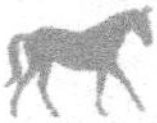	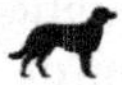
Watch	0.289	**0.746****
Near	**0.619****	0.382
Pet	**0.525***	**0.696****
Talk	**0.678****	0.382
Play	**0.633****	**0.623***
Hold	**0.540***	0.122
Hug	0.321	**0.595***
Kiss	0.087	0.293
Groom	0.413	0.145
Offer food	0.122	–
Do tricks or training	0.169	0.211
Take pictures	–	–
Decline/avoid	−0.258	−0.509
Aggressive	–	0.305
Total human-initiated HAI	**0.713****	**0.738****

Note: The table provides coefficients for correlations between individual HAIS items and positive emotion for university students in a laboratory-based EAP session. Correlations are reported separately for sessions with a horse versus a dog. Significant correlations are in bold.

$^{**}p \le 0.01$
$^{*}p < 0.05$

active behaviors that may have to do with the animal's care. These behaviors seem different from *watching*, *petting*, and *talking* to an animal, which are less active than caretaking and perhaps more casual and affiliative. In Chap. 6, I review a factor analysis of HAIS data that resulted in factors similar to the pattern seen here. This pattern of anodyne-associated behaviors could be consistent with AAI involving horses and dogs in general, or could simply reflect the HAI that occurred in this particular situation with these students and these animals. For now, the data are useful for thinking about how HAI may elicit an anodyne effect, and ways to investigate it across multiple species.

I calculated a dose–response curve for HAI and anodyne, separated by species. Because this study was posttest only, response could not be calculated as the percentage of participants whose emotion improved from pre to post, as was done with the dose–response curves shown earlier. Instead, response was defined as the percentage of participants whose positive emotion was greater than the control condition. *Greater than* was defined by the formula depicted in Fig. 4.3, where a data point (i.e., positive emotion) must be greater than the sum of the control-condition mean + 1.5 control-condition standard deviations. Since the mean positive emotion score in this control condition was 13.00 and the standard deviation was 7.85, a data point was considered a response if it was greater than 13.00 + 1.5(7.85), or 24.78.

Figure 4.4 shows the dose–response curve for these data. The overall response was greater for the dog sessions than for the horse sessions, but the shape of the curve is similar for both conditions. These data suggest an anodyne effect occurred with both species, and the dose–response relationship was similar.

$$R = X_{\text{intervention}} > [\mu_{\text{control}} + 1.5(SD_{\text{control}})]$$

$$\mu_{\text{control}} = 13.00 \qquad SD_{\text{control}} = 7.85$$

$$1.5 \times 7.85 = 11.78$$

$$13.00 + 11.78 = 24.78$$

$$R = X > 24.78$$

Fig. 4.3 Formula to calculate response for posttest-only outcome data. Formula used to calculate response, where *R* is response, *X* is a posttest positive emotion score, μ is the mean, and *SD* is the standard deviation

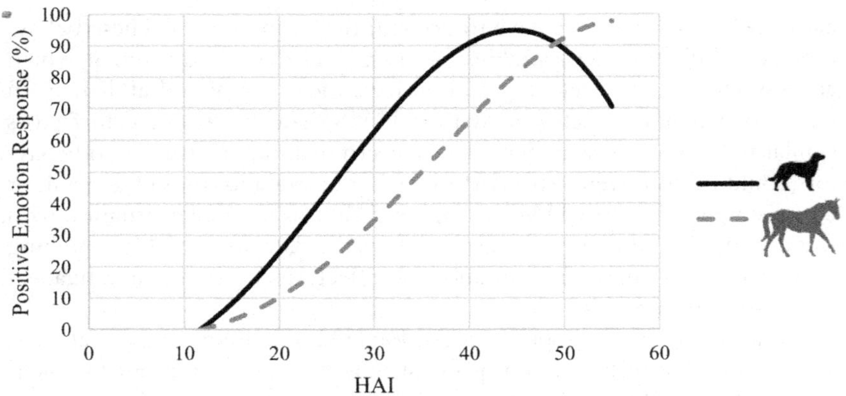

Fig. 4.4 HAI and positive emotion across species. Graph depicting the dose–response curve for total HAIS score and positive emotion, separate by sessions with a horse or a dog

Discussion

The posttest correlations in Study 1 indicate that improved mood and anxiety were associated with greater quantities of HAI. The correlations were the strongest for human-initiated behavior reported on the HAIS, compared to animal-initiated behavior. However, while some of the correlations were moderate (i.e., 0.393), others were relatively weak (i.e., 0.263). Study 2 improved upon these findings by employing a more rigorous, experimental design. Variables such as setting, facilitators, and novelty were controlled, strengthening internal validity. However, the level of control and the prescribed nature of the activity (i.e., participants were given specific instructions, processing was standardized) likely weakened the social validity of the study. These are all factors to consider in future replication.

Taken together, the correlational and experimental studies provide evidence for an anodyne effect and suggest a dose–response relationship. The number of interactions with animals was correlated with positive emotion. In the horse–dog–control study, we found an anodyne effect through experimental manipulation of HAI, keeping all other variables constant. These studies provide (1) evidence of an anodyne effect with these samples and (2) a research paradigm for comparing anodyne and other factors across species.

Implications of an Anodyne Effect

An anodyne effect could be an end in and of itself. For many activities involving animals, the objective may be to achieve just this—a temporary, perhaps superficial, increase in positive emotion or reduction in distress. Perhaps visits from animals allow patients in hospitals or nursing homes to feel a little better for a little while. Given the plethora of AAA programs in medical settings, K-12 schools, and universities and colleges (Crossman et al. 2015), an anodyne effect could have a large impact, reaching many people. Crossman (2019) argues that the flexibility and availability of HAI (e.g., no need for diagnosis or insurance) make it ideal for reducing human distress on a large scale. An anodyne effect likely impacts other, longer-term outcomes targeted by therapeutic interventions. One way the anodyne effect could impact the therapeutic process is by influencing the conditions conducive to therapeutic benefit. These conditions could include improved attention, attendance, and tolerance for the therapeutic process, as well as expanded cognitive and behavioral potential.

Attention

Gocheva et al. (2018) conducted an RCT, comparing patients with acquired brain injury who received standard versus AAT sessions. Therapy consisted of speech therapy, physiotherapy, and occupational therapy. The researchers examined the effects of AAT on concentration and attention span; these variables were measured via direct observation. Subjectively, participants reported being more alert and having better concentration during the AAT sessions.

Attendance

Calvo et al. (2016) conducted a small-scale RCT, testing AAT as an adjunct to conventional treatment for patients with schizophrenia. The AAT group improved equally to the control group on positive emotion and overall symptomatology. The AAT group showed improvement in negative symptomatology while the control group did not. In addition, the AAT group had greater attendance, with a rate of 92.9% compared to the control group's rate of 61.2%. Similarly, Beck et al. (1986) compared attendance for group therapy sessions with and without an animal. Attendance in the AAT group was more consistent, and the participants were more actively involved. Increased attendance could be due to HAI increasing one's tolerance for distress.

Tolerance

Garcia et al. (2016) examined the effect of a dog on college students' latency to escape response. Students were subjected to an aversive auditory stimulus in one of two distraction conditions—distracted by reading a book or by the presence of a dog—or a control condition with no distraction. Latency was greatest in the dog condition. Students with the dog could better tolerate the stimulus and rated the session more positively. The authors suggest dogs can positively affect the perception of aversive situations. We know that participating in some treatments can be experienced as aversive early on or during key points in the treatment regimen (e.g., Castonguay et al. 1998). Perhaps an anodyne effect can help people tolerate and persist through difficult times in treatment. In addition to affecting treatment attention, attendance, and tolerance an anodyne effect could perhaps positively impact the way people think and behave as it relates to therapeutic goals.

Cognitive and Behavioral Effects

According to the broaden-and-build theory, positive emotions broaden one's thought–action repertoire, allowing them to think more broadly and have a broader range of behaviors (Fredrickson 1998, 2001). The theory also suggests that positive emotions help build personal resources (e.g., physical skills, health, social support networks). In a test of the broaden-and-build theory, Fredrickson and Branigan (2005) had college students watch one of several short videos aimed at eliciting emotions. Videos designed to elicit positive emotions included a video on penguins or nature; those designed to elicit negative emotions included a video of a victim being taunted or a bicycle accident. There was also a neutral video designed to elicit no significant emotion—a video of sticks piling up. It was predicted that the video eliciting positive emotion would result in a global, as opposed to local, focus in visual attention and increased thought–action repertoire. This was indeed the case. Most relevant to an anodyne effect, the video showing penguins waddling, swimming, and jumping elicited feelings of amusement and happiness and those feelings were associated with the greatest broadening of attentional focus and thought–action repertoire. Can this relationship between HAI, positive emotion, and increased thought–action repertoire be applied to AAI? Can an anodyne effect broaden focus and build behavior to facilitate a therapeutic process? Research addressing this question would be useful in developing an explanatory theory on AAI.

Summary

This chapter has introduced the concept of animals as anodyne, suggesting that one way animals assist interventions is to elicit an improvement in mood or reduction in distress. This effect is related to impacting a subjective state, rather than altering a trait, symptom, or level of functioning. Although a lift in mood or decrease in subjective distress may seem minor when compared to the number of serious situations or conditions targeted by AAI (e.g., PTSD, cancer, dementia), we cannot underestimate the impact of a moment of relief on quality of life, overall well-being, or longer-term processes.

The research presented here provides preliminary evidence of an anodyne effect and illustrates research methods that may be useful in studying it further. Specifically, the analysis of behavioral HAI as it relates to an anodyne effect is important. Knowing whether certain interactive behaviors or specific quantities of HAI are potent could help us develop more effective interventions. This is important for human recipients and intervention animals. Imagine we find that petting a dog is closely associated with feeling happy and calm but grooming is not. Interventions that involve petting the dog may be more effective than ones with grooming. We could ask similar questions about time. Perhaps we find that an anodyne effect, if it will occur with a particular patient at all, will likely occur within two minutes of interaction. Then we don't need interventions to last 30 minutes. Shorter individual visits could mean a greater number of visits can be conducted, or the workload could be lessened for therapy animals and their handlers.

It should also be noted that not all AAI studies find positive outcomes, including outcomes that could be described as an anodyne effect. For example, Kaiser et al. (2002) compared the effects of a dog to a nonjudgmental "happy person" visiting residents in a nursing home. They found similar behavior, affect, and satisfaction between the two conditions. There was no difference in affect between visits from a dog versus a person. As a second example, Hartwig (2017) conducted a randomized comparison group design, comparing children who received play therapy with and without a dog. Children attended 50-minute individual sessions weekly for 10 sessions. There were significant reductions in reported anxiety and depression. However, these differences were noted in both the intervention and control conditions; there were no differences in children who did play therapy with versus without a dog.

Clearly more research is needed to determine whether an anodyne effect is a reliable AAI outcome. We might also wonder whether animals have a role in interventions *beyond* an anodyne effect. Perhaps animals can take a more active role in intervention, acting as therapeutic agents. This idea is discussed in Chap. 5.

References

American Veterinary Medical Association. (2019). Human-animal bond. Retrieved from https://www.avma.org/kb/resources/reference/human-animal-bond/pages/human-animal-bond-avma.aspx.

Aydin, N., Krueger, J. I., Fischer, J., Hahn, D., Kastenmüller, A., Frey, D., & Fischer, P. (2012). "Man's best friend": How the presence of a dog reduces mental distress after social exclusion. *Journal of Experimental Social Psychology, 48*(1), 446–449.

Barker, S. B., & Barker, R. T. (2019). Animal-assisted interventions in hospitals. In A. H. Fine (Ed.), *Handbook on animal-assisted therapy: Theoretical foundations and guidelines for practice* (5th ed., pp. 329–342). San Diego, CA: Elsevier.

Barker, S. B., & Dawson, K. S. (1998). The effects of animal-assisted therapy on anxiety ratings of hospitalized psychiatric patients. *Psychiatric Services, 49*(6), 797–801.

Barker, S. B., Pandurangi, A. K., & Best, A. M. (2003). Effects of animal-assisted therapy on patients' anxiety, fear, and depression before ECT. *The Journal of ECT, 19*(1), 38–44.

Barker, S. B., Knisely, J. S., Schubert, C. M., Green, J. D., & Ameringer, S. (2015). The effect of an animal-assisted intervention on anxiety and pain in hospitalized children. *Anthrozoös, 28*(1), 101–112.

Beck, A. M., Seraydarian, L., & Hunter, F. (1986). Use of animals in the rehabilitation of psychiatric patients. *Psychological Reports, 58*, 63–66.

Beetz, A. (2013). Socio-emotional correlates of a schooldog-teacher-team in the classroom. *Frontiers in Psychology, 4*, 886.

Berget, B., Ekeberg, Ø., Pedersen, I., & Braastad, B. O. (2011). Animal-assisted therapy with farm animals for persons with psychiatric disorders: Effects on anxiety and depression, a randomized controlled trial. *Occupational Therapy in Mental Health, 27*(1), 50–64.

Bivens, A., Leinart, D., Klontz, B., & Klontz, T. (2007). The effectiveness of equine-assisted experiential therapy: Results of an open clinical trial. *Society & Animals, 15*(3), 257–267.

Bloom, H. S., Bos, J. M., & Lee, S. W. (1999). Using cluster random assignment to measure program impacts: Statistical implications for the evaluation of education programs. *Evaluation Review, 23*(4), 445–469.

Calvo, P., Fortuny, J. R., Guzmán, S., Macías, C., Bowen, J., García, M. L., et al. (2016). Animal assisted therapy (AAT) program as a useful adjunct to conventional psychosocial rehabilitation for patients with schizophrenia: Results of a small-scale randomized controlled trial. *Frontiers in Psychology, 7*, 631.

Castonguay, L., Pincus, A., Agras, W., & Hines, C. (1998). The role of emotion in group cognitive-behavioral therapy for binge eating disorder: When things have to feel worse before they get better. *Psychotherapy Research, 8*(2), 225–238.

Chandler, C. (2017). *Animal assisted therapy in counseling* (3rd ed.). New York, NY: Routledge.

Crossman, M. (2017). Effects of interactions with animals on human psychological distress. *Journal of Clinical Psychology, 73*(7), 761–784.

Crossman, M. K. (2019). Animal-assisted activities in colleges and universities: An efficient model for reducing student stress. In A. H. Fine (Ed.), *Handbook on animal-assisted therapy: Theoretical foundations and guidelines for practice* (5th ed., pp. 207–224). San Diego, CA: Elsevier.

Crossman, M. K., Kazdin, A. E., & Knudson, K. (2015). Brief unstructured interaction with a dog reduces distress. *Anthrozoös, 28*(4), 649–659.

Drapeau, A., Marchand, A., & Beaulieu-Prévost, D. (2012). Epidemiology of psychological distress. In L. Labate (Ed.), *Mental illnesses-understanding, prediction and control* (pp. 105–134). INTECH.

Equine Assisted Growth and Learning Association. (2019). *Fundamentals of the EAGALA model: Practice untraining manual* (9th ed.). Santaquin, UT: EAGALA.

Fine, A. H. (2019a). Incorporating animal-assisted interventions into psychotherapy: Guidelines and suggestions for therapists. In A. H. Fine (Ed.), *Handbook on animal-assisted therapy: Theoretical foundations and guidelines for practice* (5th ed., pp. 207–224). San Diego, CA: Elsevier.

Fine, A. H. (2019b). *Handbook on animal-assisted therapy: Theoretical foundations and guidelines for practice* (5th ed.). San Diego, CA: Elsevier.

Fournier, A. K., Berry, T. D., Letson, E. A., & Chanen, R. (2016). The human-animal interaction scale: Development and evaluation. *Anthrozoös, 29*(3), 455–467.

Fournier, A. K., Berry, T. D., Letson, E. A., Laitala, J., Proels, L., & Kavanagh, K. (in press). The anodyne-agent model: A framework for understanding animal-assisted intervention. *Human-Animal Interaction Bulletin.*

Fournier, A. K., Letson, E. A., Berry, T. D., & Pasiuk, E. (2018). Human-animal interaction and metaphor in equine-assisted psychotherapy: Empirical support for the EAGALA model. *Human-Animal Interaction Bulletin, 6*(1), 47–63.

Fredrickson, B. L. (1998). What good are positive emotions? *Review of General Psychology, 2*(3), 300.

Fredrickson, B. L. (2001). The role of positive emotions in positive psychology: The broaden-and-build theory of positive emotions. *American Psychologist, 56*(3), 218.

Fredrickson, B. L. (2004). The broaden-and-build theory of positive emotions. *Philosophical Transactions of the Royal Society B: Biological Sciences, 359*(1449), 1367.

Fredrickson, B. L., & Branigan, C. (2005). Positive emotions broaden the scope of attention and thought-action repertoires. *Cognition & Emotion, 19*(3), 313–332. https://doi.org/10.1080/02699930441000238.

Galanakis, M., Stalikas, A., Pezirkianidis, C., & Karakasidou, I. (2016). Reliability and validity of the modified differential emotions scale (mDES) in a Greek sample. *Psychology, 7*(1), 101.

Garcia, G., Sodré, L., Zaine, I., & Domeniconi, C. (2016). Influence of dog presence on the tolerance and evaluation of aversive stimulation. *Pet Behavior Science, 2*, 16–23.

Gocheva, V., Hund-Georgiadis, M., & Hediger, K. (2018). Effects of animal-assisted therapy on concentration and attention span in patients with acquired brain injury: A randomized controlled trial. *Neuropsychology, 32*(1), 54.

Grajfoner, D., Harte, E., Potter, L., & McGuigan, N. (2017). The effect of dog-assisted intervention on student well-being, mood, and anxiety. *International Journal of Environmental Research and Public Health, 14*(5), 483.

Hartwig, E. K. (2017). Building solutions in youth: Evaluation of the human–animal resilience therapy intervention. *Journal of Creativity in Mental Health, 12*(4), 468–481.

Hoffmann, A. O., Lee, A. H., Wertenauer, F., Ricken, R., Jansen, J. J., Gallinat, J., & Lang, U. E. (2009). Dog-assisted intervention significantly reduces anxiety in hospitalized patients with major depression. *European Journal of Integrative Medicine, 1*(3), 145–148.

Holcomb, R., Jendro, C., Weber, B., & Nahan, U. (1997). Use of an aviary to relieve depression in elderly males. *Anthrozoös, 10*(1), 32–36.

Kaiser, L., Spence, L. J., McGavin, L., Struble, L., & Keilman, L. (2002). A dog and a "happy person" visit nursing home residents. *Western Journal of Nursing Research, 24*(6), 671–683.

Kaplan, D. M., Smith, T., & Coons, J. (1995). A validity study of the subjective unit of discomfort (SUD) score. *Measurement and Evaluation in Counseling and Development, 27*(4), 195–199.

Kern-Godal, A., Brenna, I. H., Kogstad, N., Arnevik, E. A., & Ravndal, E. (2016). Contribution of the patient–horse relationship to substance use disorder treatment: Patients' experiences. *International Journal of Qualitative Studies on Health and Well-Being, 11*(1), 31636.

Kreivinienė, B., & Perttula, J. (2014). Dolphin assisted therapy: Innovative learning for children with disabilities. *Education in a Changing Society, 1*, 90–98.

Merriam-Webster. (2019). Anodyne. Retrieved from https://www.merriam-webster.com/dictionary/anodyne.

Muela, A., Balluerka, N., Amiano, N., Caldentey, M., Aliri, J., & Muela, A. (2017). Animal-assisted psychotherapy for young people with behavioural problems in residential care. *Clinical Psychology & Psychotherapy, 24*(6), O1485–O1494.

Murthy, R., Bearman, G., Brown, S., Bryant, K., Chinn, R., Hewlett, A., et al. (2015). Animals in healthcare facilities: Recommendations to minimize potential risks. *Infection Control & Hospital Epidemiology, 36*(5), 495–516.

Oliva, V. N. L. S., Albuquerque, V. B., Silva, E. Y. T., Yamamoto, K. C. M., Costa, K. N., Silva, M. L. M., et al. (2010). Institutionalized elderly and animal assisted activities (AAA). *Revista Ciência em Extensão, 6*(2), 15–31.

Rothbaum, B. O., Astin, M. C., & Marsteller, F. (2005). Prolonged exposure versus eye movement desensitization and reprocessing (EMDR) for PTSD rape victims. *Journal of Traumatic Stress, 18*(6), 607–616.

Stewart, L. A., Dispenza, F., Parker, L., Chang, C. Y., & Cunnien, T. (2014). A pilot study assessing the effectiveness of an animal-assisted outreach program. *Journal of Creativity in Mental Health, 9*(3), 332–345.

Turner, D. C. (2017). A review of over three decades of research on cat-human and human-cat interactions and relationships. *Behavioural Processes, 141*, 297–304.

Wolpe, J. (1990). *The practice of behavior therapy*. Oxford: Pergamon.

Wood, W., Fields, B., Rose, M., & McLure, M. (2017). Animal-assisted therapies and dementia: A systematic mapping review using the lived environment life quality (LELQ) model. *American Journal of Occupational Therapy, 71*(5), 1–10.

CHAPTER 5

Animals as Intervention Agents

Abstract This chapter describes a second role animals may play in assisting intervention—a therapeutic agent. The animal-assisted intervention (AAI) literature describes investigation of a variety of outcomes (e.g., reduction of symptoms, improvements in behavior, changes in psychosocial constructs), and suggests potential theories to explain these outcomes (e.g., social support, attachment). I argue that the variety of outcomes is because of the innumerable goals targeted by AAI, and that an overarching construct can be helpful in framing the animal's role in achieving any of these goals. Animals will be discussed as agents within the intervention process. Although not described in this way, the literature sometimes refers to the animal's role as an agent or substitute. The chapter will cite literature on animal characteristics that make them potential agents (e.g., capacity for self-willed action, nonthreatening, unconditional positive regard) and describe research identifying animals as intervention agents. The roles of anodyne and agent are combined to introduce the anodyne-agent model, a framework for understanding the role of the therapy animal in AAI.

Keywords Agent • Animal-assisted intervention • Psychotherapy • Equine-assisted psychotherapy • Eagala

A. K. Fournier, *Animal-Assisted Intervention*,
https://doi.org/10.1007/978-3-030-32972-3_5

To date, the animal-assisted intervention (AAI) literature describes investigation of a variety of outcomes (e.g., reduction of symptoms, improvements in behavior, changes in psychosocial constructs), and suggests potential theories to explain these outcomes. Theoretical explanations include, but are not limited to, activation of the social response mechanism which increases reward hormones such as oxytocin and dopamine (Odendaal 2000; Odendaal and Meintjes 2003), buffering of the stress response through social support (Garrity and Stallones 1998; Serpell 1996), distraction from aversive experiences and mental states (Barker et al. 2015), and an innate predisposition to attend to living organisms (i.e., biophilia) (Wilson 1984). Each of these theories is important in guiding AAI investigation. However, the number of outcomes measured in AAI can leave practitioners and researchers confused as to what AAI is and which outcomes to measure. Chapter 4 discussed the anodyne effect, which wherein one of the ways animals facilitate interventions is by reducing negative emotions and/or increasing positive emotions. In other words, animals help people feel better (e.g., calm, soothed). In this chapter, I present another overarching construct to help us see AAI outcome in a broader context. We can think of animals serving as *agents* in the intervention process, whatever that intervention might be. The variety of different AAI outcomes (e.g., depressive or anxiety symptoms, social behavior, self-efficacy) can be explained by the innumerable therapeutic goals targeted by interventions.

Put most simply, an agent is one who is authorized to act for or in place of another (Merriam-Webster 2019a). Although not labeled as such, the animal-assisted therapy (AAT) literature often describes animals serving as agents in the intervention process, substituting for important others, a construct, a situation, or the environment at large. This is true in animal-assisted mental- and physical-health intervention.

Animals as Agents in Mental-Health Intervention

In Aydin et al.'s (2011) finding that an unfamiliar dog helped socially excluded participants, they suggest dogs serve as stand-ins for humans, mediating social isolation. Corson and O'Leary Corson (1980) indicate therapy dogs helped with loneliness by serving as communication mediators, providing nonthreatening nonverbal communication. Animals are frequently described as helping people by offering social support (e.g., Serpell 1996; Serpell et al. 2017). In this case, the human may need positive social interaction or positive relationships; animals can serve as the agent of interaction or relation, rather than or in addition to a human. In psychotherapy, it is suggested that animals serve as subjects onto which thoughts and feelings can be projected (e.g., Wells et al. 1997); this allows the client to identify and work on therapeutic issues with or through the animal. In addition, the literature suggests animals help people learn appropriate social behavior, modeling desirable or undesirable behavior (e.g., Mueller et al. 2019), or serving as a social other to interact with and provide feedback (Brooks 2001).

Human–animal relational theory is a theory to explain animal-assisted counseling (Chandler 2018). The theory suggests bringing an animal into the counseling process increases the relational dynamics and thus increases the potential for *significant relational moments*. These relational moments can be between any of the counseling-session participants—between the client and the therapy animal, the client and the counselor, the therapy animal and the counselor, or between all three. Chandler suggests that relational moments provide opportunity for clients to identify and work on therapeutic issues. The studies reviewed here describe animals serving as attachment figures, social mediators, or sources of social support. Rather than developing separate theories to explain each of these roles, we can think of animals serving as agents in the intervention process to meet client needs, whichever needs are being targeted (e.g., attachment, social connection, social support).

For instance, including an animal in animal-assisted psychotherapy does not determine the diagnosis, treatment goals, or treatment plan; and it does not determine the overall mechanism of change. It provides an alternate method for *implementing* the treatment. For example, psychotherapy for depression, whether including an animal or not, is targeted at reducing depressive symptoms and improving functioning. Including an animal in the treatment (i.e., animal-assisted psychotherapy) is a means of delivery, or *modality*. The animal may serve as a substitute for the practitioner, significant others, important constructs (e.g., goals, challenges) or the world as it relates to symptoms and functioning. This framework can also apply to interventions targeting physical symptoms and function.

Animals as Agents in Physical-Health Intervention

Animals are involved in interventions in a variety of allied-health fields, including physical therapy and occupational therapy. According to the American Occupational Therapy Association (2019), occupational therapy encourages rehabilitation in people who have experienced illness or injury, through performance of everyday activities (i.e., occupations). Velde et al. (2005) analyzed three qualitative case studies of AAT in occupational therapy, analyzing patient and practitioner perceptions. Therapists indicated that patients benefit physically when an animal is included, reporting that patients had greater range of motion, sensory modulation and interpretation, and greater tolerance for painful physical activities. For example, clients in need of intervention to improve range of motion could be given tasks to do with or to a therapy dog (e.g., walk with the dog, brush the dog) that facilitate increased range of motion. In this case, the dog becomes an agent in the occupational therapy targeting range of motion. These authors also discussed animal caretaking as fulfilling an important lost role—that of caretaker. In addition, the dog was credited with facilitating communication with family members. In each of these examples, occupational therapy targets a goal—increasing range of motion, serving as caretaker or family member—and the animal is an agent in achieving that goal.

Abate et al. (2011) studied a canine-assisted physical-therapy intervention for chronic heart-failure patients. The target of the intervention was increased ambulation (i.e., walking) as it is associated with better outcomes and reduced hospital stay. The physical-therapy refusal rate of a sample of 69 hospitalized patients was compared with a 537-patient historical population. The refusal rate in the historical population was 28.1% while the canine-assisted rate was 7.2%. In addition, number of steps walked for the canine-assisted patients was almost double that of the historical comparison group. In this situation, the goal of the intervention was for patients to walk. The dog served as an agent by providing them a novel walking partner.

Yap et al. (2017) surveyed medical staff of a children's hospital on their attitudes, beliefs, and concerns surrounding AAT for children. The participants worked with children diagnosed with cerebral palsy, autism spectrum disorders, and acquired brain injury. The staff identified several ways AAT could benefit patients. Regarding physical-health outcomes, these medical professionals indicated a dog could assist with "physical rehabilitation including gait control, encouraging movement and the training of high-level functional skills in addition to improving coordination and muscle building" (Yap et al. 2017, p. 48).

Why Animals?

One could ask why animals should be considered intervention agents. What are the qualities or characteristics of animals that allow them to be effective agents? Practitioners and researchers often discuss this issue, mentioning animals in general, as well as particular species. One basic characteristic that gives animals the capacity to serve in this role is that animals have agency. Beyond a mere prop in the therapeutic space, animals have agency with which to engage.

Animal Agency

We can think of agency as the capacity, condition, or state of acting or of exerting power (Merriam-Webster 2019b). Animals have a degree of agency that allows them to assist in interventions. Animal agency is addressed in the literature from both philosophical and sociological perspectives. While some argue that agency requires the animal to perform an action that alters their circumstances within a social structure (Carter and Charles 2013), others define agency simply as the capacity for self-willed action (Irvine 2008; Jerolmack 2005). The latter definition is helpful in discussing AAI; animals have the capacity for autonomous action (e.g., a therapy animal moves away from a client) and intervention can occur through that action (e.g., client interprets the animal's movement as rejection, identifies a thought pattern). While there is growing literature confirming animal cognition and sentience (e.g., Marino and Colvin 2015), these characteristics are not assumed nor necessary for animals to serve as intervention agents. Instead, animal agency as I am describing it here, is limited to the animal's self-initiated observable behavior, which a client can interpret and respond to. Examination of animal agency supports this notion—that animals can impact the situation through autonomous action without assuming intention (Shaw 2013). Although the human recipient of an AAI may *perceive* the therapy animal to have particular thoughts, feelings, or intentions about them or the situation; any focus on internal experience as part of the therapeutic process would be that of the *human* not the *animal*. The literature provides some guidance as it relates to animal agency in general and associated characteristics.

Animal Characteristics

Theories on the mechanisms of change in AAI "focus on the supposedly unique intrinsic attributes of animals that appear to contribute to therapy. Others emphasize the value of animals as living instruments that can be used to affect positive changes in patients' self-concept and behavior through the patients' acquisition of various skills and acceptance of personal agency and responsibility" (Kruger and Serpell 2006, p. 26). Thus, two factors—animal attributes and working relationship—are identified in a variety of potential theoretical explanations. However, perhaps it is *because* of animals' unique attributes that they *can* serve as agents in working relationships resulting in positive change. For example, Myers (1998) suggests that animals can provide social support to humans because they elicit positive affect and do not pose a threat. Chandler suggests that an animal's stress response system allows them to detect emotional distress for humans during interactions (Chandler 2017). There is significant evidence that we attend to animals when they are present (Buttelmann and Römpke 2014; Havey et al. 2014). Whether based in our biology (Wilson 1984) or our learning history (Brickel 2016), many people are drawn to animals. Because of or in addition to this, their nonverbal, nonthreatening, in-the-moment presence makes them potential agents in the therapeutic process.

Species

To date, there is discussion of species-specific characteristics that coincide with therapeutic potential, but the suppositions have not been borne out through research. Horses and dogs, being popular therapy animals, are sometimes discussed as effective therapy agents in different ways. In a report by the Canadian Agency for Drugs and Technologies in Health (2012), dogs were described as effective with people who experienced trauma and had dementia, while horses were thought to be most effective with children who had attention deficit hyperactivity disorder (ADHD) or experienced family violence. Practitioners attest to horses' ability to mirror human emotions and body language. This, in combination with their size, can reportedly provide instant, unbiased feedback to the client (Vidrine et al. 2002; Bivens et al. 2007). On the other hand, dogs, being predatory animals, show a different set of useful behaviors. For example, dogs were shown to have more interest in interacting with humans than horses. Dogs are also more likely to make eye contact with humans, which may strengthen the emotional bond and facilitate release of oxytocin in both the dog and the human (Nagasawa et al. 2015). Following are two examples of animals—dogs and horses—serving as agents.

Dogs as Agents in Healthy Expression of Masculinity

The PenPals research discussed in Chap. 1 (Fournier et al. 2007) can provide an example of dogs serving as agents for prison inmates. The data were examined within the context of masculinity in the prison setting (Fournier 2016). Self-reported interactions and experiences were provided by 102 inmates who had applied to work in the PenPals program but were not yet enrolled. They completed the Human–Animal Interaction Scale (HAIS), reporting their interactions with program dogs over the past week. Even though they were not in the program, they reported a great deal of interaction with the PenPals dogs. Human-initiated behaviors included casual behaviors like *watching* and *petting* the dogs, but also included more close, intimate behaviors like *holding*, *hugging*, or *kissing* the dogs. The inmates participated in focus groups, discussing their impressions of the program. Comments suggested interactions with the dogs helped them feel more human, giving them a sense of accomplishment, freedom, and purpose. Analysis of the HAIS scores and comments suggested interactions with dogs allowed for healthy expression of masculinity, which is limited in prison settings. For example, caring for the unwanted shelter dogs allowed them to enact empathy, training dogs to prevent euthanasia allowed for heroism, and playing with the dogs allowed for action-oriented relating. Essentially, the dogs served as agents for the expression of healthy masculinity, as opposed to the toxic masculinity (Kupers 2001) that otherwise permeates male correctional facilities (Amato 2012; Phillips 2001). This role of the human–animal bond in gender expression is not confined to the prison environment. For more on the role of dogs in male gender roles and expression of masculinity, see Blazina and Kogan (2016). Next, two empirical studies are discussed in which horses served as therapeutic agents.

Horses as Agents in Psychotherapy and Learning

In Chap. 4, a study was described in which 112 adults attended one or more equine-assisted psychotherapy (EAP) sessions and reported on human–animal interaction (HAI) and distress. In addition to the anodyne effect already discussed, the second part of the study involves an exploration of the role of the horses in assisting with an outcome that could have longer-term effects—psychosocial learning. The study is described in greater detail elsewhere (Fournier et al. 2018) and summarized here in the context of animals as therapeutic agents.

Horses as Agents Through Metaphor

Much of the method was mentioned in Chap. 3 when discussing anodyne. Following an Eagala-model EAP session, participants completed the HAIS and Subjective Units of Distress Scale (SUDS). In addition, they rated items on metaphor and psychosocial learning. Metaphor is an important concept in the Eagala model (Eagala 2015; Notgrass and Pettinelli 2015) and is mentioned in other equine-assisted work (e.g., Gilbert 2013; Lujan 2012; Schultz et al. 2007), as well as other AAI literature (O'Callaghan, O'Callaghan 2008). Metaphor can be defined as "a device for seeing something in terms of something else" (Burke 1941, p. 421). In AAI, an animal can serve as a metaphor for something or someone else. Clinical cases describe horses as metaphors for diagnoses, such as drug addiction, or relationship constructs like trust and communication (Letson 2012). Our team gathered data on whether horses served as metaphors in EAP and if those metaphors were related to therapeutic outcome (i.e., psychosocial learning).

Metaphor and psychosocial learning were recorded on the Metaphor Record, a self-report instrument designed to gather quantitative and qualitative data on the content of an intervention session (Letson and Fournier 2017). Clients are asked to rate their agreement with statements that (1) the animals in the session represented something in their life, and (2) they learned something about themselves or their life. A rating of 0 indicated they did not agree with the statement at all; 10 indicated they agreed completely. Next to their rating for each item, participants were asked to provide written comments explaining their ratings. These written comments were analyzed following the constant comparative method (Brunner 2004); three researchers independently read the comments and identified themes. Researchers discussed, settled on a number of themes, and then categorized each written response into one of the themes. This process was followed for the themes on horses as metaphors and psychosocial learning.[1]

Participants reported learning about their own strengths and weaknesses (34.0%, $n = 18$), identified personal relationship patterns (28.3%, $n = 15$), became aware of their emotions (17.0%, $n = 9$), came to acknowledge or accept something about themselves or their life (9.4%, $n = 5$), and set goals or identified interests (7.5%, $n = 4$). These are valuable outcomes

[1] Of the 112 participants, the numbers who provided written comments on metaphor and psychosocial learning was 53 and 51. All comments were categorized by two independent researchers; interrater agreement was 88%.

and are helpful in understanding what the effects of EAP could be. But can we connect these outcomes to the *animals* in this intervention? Did the horses serve as agents in the therapeutic process?

Participants overwhelmingly reported the horses represented something in their life: 87.6% of respondents reported some level of agreement with the statement; the mean level of agreement was 6.02 ($SD = 3.10$). And what did the horses represent? Client comments indicated the horses represented a feeling or state (28.1%, $n = 16$), family or friends (19.3%, $n = 11$), a relationship or relationship construct (14.0%, $n = 8$), challenges or barriers (8.8%, $n = 5$), life lessons (12.3%, $n = 7$), and themselves (10.5%, $n = 6$).

Labeling horses as something else transforms them into agents through which clients can work on therapeutic goals. In the Eagala model specifically, "having clients spend time developing relationships with the horses begins revealing the dynamics they employ and the types of relationships they have with others, things, or themselves" (Thomas and Lytle 2016, p. 151). For example, a client working on assertiveness at work can label a horse as their boss or coworker, identify their thought and behavior patterns around assertiveness through interactions with the horse, and try out new ways of thinking and asserting themselves with the horse before applying it in the workplace.

Psychosocial learning was positively correlated with human-initiated HAI, $r\ (81) = 0.39$, $p < 0.001$; horse-initiated HAI, $r\ (88) = 0.29$, $p = 0.006$; and total HAI $r\ (81) = 0.41$, $p < 0.001$. Greater interaction with the horses was associated with greater learning about self. To test for a relationship between interacting with the horses (i.e., HAIS scores), metaphor, and psychosocial learning, we conducted a mediation analysis, testing whether the relationship between HAI and psychosocial learning was mediated by metaphor. In other words, did HAI impact psychosocial learning *through* metaphor (i.e., through labeling and engaging with horses as something else)?

The mediation model was confirmed.[2] When metaphor ratings were entered into the equation, the relationship between HAI and learning was no longer significant. It seems that for these clients, human–horse interaction impacted learning through metaphor. We can also look at this within the larger context of psychotherapy.

[2] For statistical information, see original publication (Fournier et al. 2018).

Intersection with Traditional Training Models

As mentioned before, practitioners in AAT most often are first trained in their medical or mental-health field. For example, the mental-health professional in Eagala-model EAP must hold a license to practice (Eagala 2015; Notgrass and Pettinelli 2015), meaning they must hold a graduate degree in a mental-health field (e.g., counseling, clinical psychology, social work) and have completed state requirements for licensure. Then the clinician must complete training or certification in Eagala-model EAP as a treatment *modality*. As another example, the International Institute for Animal-Assisted Play Therapy (IIAAPT) requires practitioners to hold a master's or doctoral degree in a mental-health, allied-health, or education field; hold a mental-health license to practice; be credentialed in play therapy; and then be certified in animal-assisted play therapy (IIAAPT 2018; Sori and Hughes 2014; VanFleet and Faa-Thompson 2017). Both examples require mental-health education and training before certification in delivery of the animal-assisted modality. Because mental-health training can follow any of several psychotherapy models or orientations (e.g., psychodynamic, cognitive-behavioral, humanistic), mental-health specialists practicing EAP may come from a variety of different therapeutic orientations.

Treatment Modality within Therapeutic Orientation
Therapeutic orientation is defined by the American Psychological Association (APA) as "an organized set of assumptions or preferences for given theories that provides a counselor or clinician with a conceptual framework for understanding a client's needs and formulating a rationale for specific interventions" (APA 2018). The clinician's therapeutic orientation guides their interpretation of client behavior, suggests the etiology of problems, shapes treatment goals, and prescribes methods used to achieve those goals.

Chandler et al. (2010) addressed this issue, integrating literature on AAT and counseling theory. They described ways in which each of several therapeutic orientations can be consistent with AAT techniques (e.g., reflecting on client's relationship with the therapy animal) and intentions (e.g., building rapport). For example, they suggest a friendly therapy animal with an accepting nature can contribute to a feeling of unconditional positive regard and a safe therapeutic environment, two important factors in person-centered therapy (Rogers 1979). Within psychoanalytic psychotherapy or counseling, AAT could be useful in identifying unconscious wishes and drives, through transference of feelings onto the animal as a transitional object (Chandler et al. 2010). Similarly, Karol (2007) described the EAP process from a psychodynamic perspective. Six aspects of EAP were discussed as conducive to therapeutic work, including the experience of being in relationship with the horse and the therapeutic relationship with the clinician. Karol states that EAP is a rich setting for cultivating metaphor, which can connect the client's internal and external worlds (Karol 2007). The latter is key in Eagala-model EAP, given the emphasis on metaphor as a critical aspect for client interpretations of the external world (e.g., horse behavior) to raise awareness of their internal world (e.g., thoughts, emotions, patterns of behavior). These authors also discuss AAT intersecting with a cognitive-behavioral orientation, suggesting the relationship between the client and the therapy animal can be helpful in identifying irrational beliefs and self-defeating behavior.

Eagala-model EAP is described as a treatment "modality" (Notgrass and Pettinelli 2015) and used as an adjunct to other forms of treatment (Brandt 2013). Figure 5.1 illustrates a theoretical conceptualization of Eagala-model EAP in the context of therapeutic orientation. Therapeutic

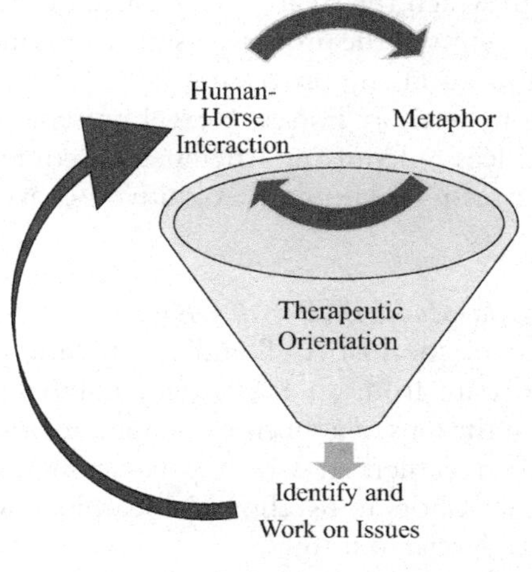

Fig. 5.1 Conceptualization of Eagala-model EAP intersecting with therapeutic orientation. Depicts Eagala-model EAP as a modality involving human–horse interaction and application of metaphors. Session content can be filtered through the clinician's therapeutic orientation to identify and work on issues

orientation assumes specific psychological mechanisms of change and provides a framework for organizing treatment goals and objectives and interpreting client behavior. Eagala-model EAP is a set of practices meant to allow clients to become aware of and address therapeutic issues through metaphor, which can be interpreted through the lens of the clinician's orientation. Just as metaphor is a vehicle for uncovering and addressing psychological issues, Eagala-model EAP can be a vehicle for carrying out psychotherapy objectives within a variety of therapeutic orientations.

For example, a cognitive-behavioral psychotherapist treating a client for anxiety, whether including an animal or not, will likely help the client identify and restructure maladaptive thoughts (e.g., something bad is going to happen) and behaviors (e.g., avoidance) related to anxiety (Beck and Beck 1995). The *goal* is anxiety reduction; the therapeutic *mechanism of change* is identification and restructuring of maladaptive thoughts and behaviors. On the other hand, a psychodynamic psychotherapist treating the same client might help them identify and process unconscious trauma or pain from childhood that is driving maladaptive patterns (Quatman 2015). The goal is the same—anxiety reduction. The mechanism of change is identifying and processing unconscious childhood trauma rather than restructuring present-day thoughts and feelings. AAT can be seen as a *modality* through which the treatment is carried out, with one or more animals serving as agents in the process. Using an equine-assisted modality would mean identification and processing occur, at least in part, through interactions with one or more horses. Next, I present an empirical investigation of these ideas, identifying therapeutic content resulting from Eagala-model EAP sessions within the cognitive-behavioral therapy (CBT) framework.

Intersection of Eagala-Model EAP with CBT

To address the intersection of AAT and therapeutic orientation empirically, we analyzed data from an EAP client database, examining client comments through the lens of a specific therapeutic orientation. Using the same data described earlier, in which participant comments indicated horses served as metaphors in psychosocial learning, we analyzed for the development of CBT-related insight.

Participant responses to the question, what, if anything, did you learn about yourself or your life? were analyzed within a cognitive-behavioral framework. Specifically, each comment ($n = 53$) was rated as a new awareness of (a) thoughts, (b) feelings, or (c) behavior. Comments were rated by two independent researchers, with an agreement rate of 98%. As Fig. 5.2 shows, comments most frequently addressed thoughts (58.5%, $n = 31$). Some comments indicated a realization of a *maladaptive* thought (e.g., "I thought I was a failure because of the events in my life."). Some of the comments seemed to suggest a *restructured* thought (e.g., "I have growth by seeing my trauma is sort of a gift"), and others suggested the client came to hold a more optimistic outlook (e.g., "I will make it," "I can do it"). Comments indicated an awareness of behavior in 32.1% of the responses ($n = 17$). These included becoming aware of *maladaptive* behaviors (e.g., "I always put myself last") and identifying *aspirational* behaviors (e.g., "I should take more time to relax and enjoy life"). Feelings were the least frequent (9.4%, $n = 2$) and tended to relate to the identification of negative emotions (e.g., "I'm stuck with anxiety").[3] To further explore the process and outcome variables, a one-way ANOVA was calculated, comparing HAIS and SUDS scores across clients who reported thoughts, feelings, and behaviors. There were no significant differences detected, p values > 0.05.

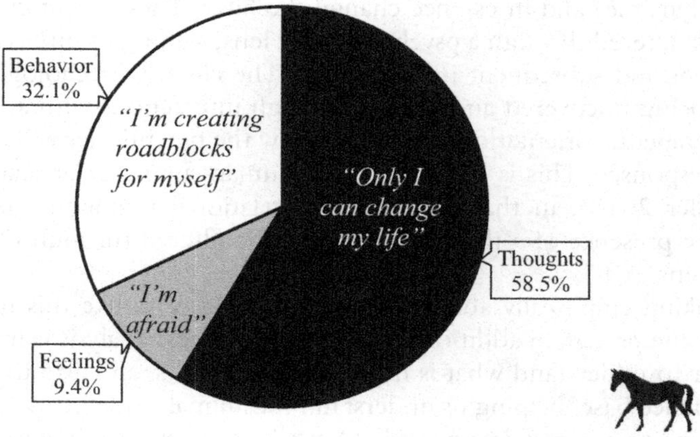

Fig. 5.2 Increased awareness following equine-assisted psychotherapy and learning session. Graph showing the percentage of clients reporting increased awareness of thoughts, feelings, and behaviors following sessions in equine-assisted growth and learning. Sample comments are paraphrased for illustration

[3] Comments from three participants consisted of descriptions of the session and could not be coded as indicating an awareness of thoughts, feelings, or behaviors.

Because of the small sample size, we cannot say that these findings are typical for the population at large. They simply represent what these clients experienced and shared following an EAP session, and how their comments were perceived by our research team. Sharing them here provides an example of how engagement in an AAI can occur within a traditional treatment method and one way to gather data on the process. Within the context of CBT, these identified thoughts, feelings, and behaviors are part of the treatment process in which clients identify maladaptive patterns and make adjustments toward more adaptive patterns. In traditional psychotherapy, thoughts, feelings, and behaviors would be uncovered and restructured through talking with the therapist, recalling life situations, and processing real-world experiences through homework assignments. In EAP, identification, restructuring, and application occurs in the session with a live animal. Again, the treatment goals and mechanism of change are the same, but the way the treatment is carried out differs. This is an example of a specific modality (Eagala-model EAP) in the context of a specific therapeutic orientation—CBT. Looking again at Fig. 5.1, we could apply a different psychotherapeutic orientation (e.g., psychodynamic) and in essence change the filter. These client comments could be filtered through a psychodynamic lens, leading to different interpretations and subsequent interventions. The client's psychological process is being uncovered and revised through interactions with an animal. The therapeutic orientation determines how the practitioner will interpret client responses. This is consistent with human–animal relational theory (Chandler 2018), in that the increased relational moments that result from the presence of a therapy animal can be filtered through the counselor's lens.

Thinking empirically about AAI, we can find ways like this to gather data on the *process*, in addition to outcomes. Process analysis is important in order to understand what is happening for clients, and also to develop the evidence base, helping us understand the animal's role in an AAI. I am suggesting that in the data provided here, horses served as agents. Clients engaged with horses and through those interactions identified ways they were thinking, feeling, and behaving. From there, interventions can be applied in which the client applies new thoughts and behaviors with the horses. For practitioners, it may be useful to gather this type of data over time for an individual client or therapy animal. Doing so could help you better understand a client process and how it may or may not relate to their interactions with the therapy animal(s).

Remember that reported mood and anxiety data from this study were discussed in Chap. 4 as evidence of the anodyne effect. The horses in these sessions may have elicited an anodyne effect and served as intervention agents by providing a vehicle through which to enact the therapeutic process. The literature reviewed earlier, discussing animals serving as agents in mental- or physical-health intervention, also mentioned the animal's role in emotional outcomes. For example, Yap and colleagues mentioned animals serving as calming agents that can help with emotion regulation (Yap et al. 2017). Abate et al. (2011) described patients' increased enjoyment and satisfaction with walks accompanied by a dog. Velde et al. (2005) concluded that animals can, among other things, improve a person's happiness and provide companionship. These emotional outcomes in combination with the animal's role as agent in the therapeutic process illustrate two potential roles for the therapy animal: eliciting an anodyne effect and serving as an intervention agent. These two overarching constructs can be combined to form a framework for thinking empirically about AAIs.

The Anodyne-Agent Model

The anodyne-agent model is a framework suggesting animals play two roles in AAI: (1) eliciting an anodyne effect and/or (2) serving as an agent in the therapeutic process. The framework, depicted in Fig. 5.3, can be useful in summarizing previous research and guiding questions for future research. The line directly from HAI to distress reduction is a representation of the anodyne effect discussed in Chap. 4. An example could be a dog and their handler providing brief unstructured visits to hospital patients, and the hospital patients experiencing reduced distress. In AAIs such as this, the animal may have just one role—eliciting anodyne. The intervention recipient feels soothed and that is the only outcome.

Referring again to Fig. 5.3, there is also a line from the intervention (e.g., psychotherapy, occupational therapy) to the outcome (e.g., reduced symptoms, improved functioning), indicating the intervention has a direct effect on the targeted outcome. The line from HAI to the intervention–outcome line represents an agent effect, in which interaction with an animal moderates, or alters, the effect of the intervention on the outcome. In psychological models such as this, a *moderator* is an independent variable that changes the nature of the relationship between other variables (APA 2019). Involving an animal in an occupational therapy intervention alters how the intervention causes or elicits the outcome. There could be additional lines

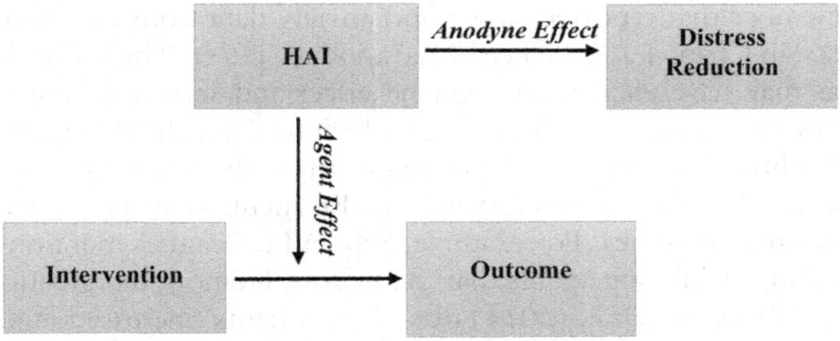

Fig. 5.3 The anodyne-agent model. The model identifies two roles for the animal in AAI. An anodyne effect is illustrated with the line from HAI to distress reduction. The line from HAI to the intervention–outcome line suggests HAI moderates the relationship between the intervention and outcome

from distress reduction to other variables that eventually lead to outcome. As mentioned in Chap. 4, it is possible that the distress reduction of the anodyne effect could increase attendance or attention to an intervention which would impact the outcome. For simplicity, these variables/relationships are not included. Rather, this illustration focuses on two roles of HAI: a direct effect on distress reduction and a moderating effect on the relationship between the intervention and the outcome.

My team and I plan to follow up this research with larger, more diverse samples. Given the great number of practitioners and therapy animals providing AAI, there is the potential for large-scale data collection, which is necessary to better understand the AAI process and develop the evidence base. In Chap. 6, I suggest applying the citizen-science approach to AAI, employing AAI practitioners to think empirically and contribute to the research.

References

Abate, S. V., Zucconi, M., & Boxer, B. A. (2011). Impact of canine-assisted ambulation on hospitalized chronic heart failure patients' ambulation outcomes and satisfaction: A pilot study. *Journal of Cardiovascular Nursing, 26*(3), 224–230.

Amato, F. J. (2012). The relationship of violence to gender role conflict and conformity to masculine norms in a forensic sample. *The Journal of Men's Studies, 20*(3), 187–208.

American Occupational Therapy Association. (2019). *About occupational therapy*. Retrieved from https://www.aota.org/About-Occupational-Therapy.aspx.

American Psychological Association. (2018). *Theoretical orientation*. APA dictionary of psychology. Retrieved from https://dictionary.apa.org/theoretical-orientation.

American Psychological Association. (2019). *Moderator*. APA dictionary of psychology. Retrieved from https://dictionary.apa.org/moderator.

Aydin, N., Krueger, J. I., Fischer, J., Hahn, D., Kastenmüller, A., Frey, D., & Fischer, P. (2011). "Man's best friend": how the presence of a dog reduces mental distress after social exclusion. *Journal of Experimental Social Psychology, 48*(1), 446–449. https://doi.org/10.1016/j.jesp.2011.09.011.

Barker, S. B., Knisely, J. S., Schubert, C. M., Green, J. D., & Ameringer, S. (2015). The effect of an animal-assisted intervention on anxiety and pain in hospitalized children. *Anthrozoös, 28*(1), 101–112. https://doi.org/10.2752/089279315X14129350722091.

Beck, J. S., & Beck, A. T. (1995). *Cognitive therapy: Basics and beyond*. New York: Guilford Press.

Bivens, A., Leinart, D., Klontz, B., & Klontz, T. (2007). The effectiveness of equine-assisted experiential therapy: Results of an open clinical trial. *Society & Animals, 15*(3), 257–267.

Blazina, C., & Kogan, L. (2016). *Men and their dogs: A new understanding of man's best friend*. AG Switzerland: Springer.

Brandt, C. (2013). Equine-facilitated psychotherapy as a complementary treatment intervention. *The Practitioner Scholar: Journal of Counseling and Professional Psychology, 2*(1), 23–42.

Brickel, C. M. (2016). Initiation and maintenance of the human-animal bond: Familial roles from a learning perspective. In *Pets and the family* (pp. 31–48). Routledge.

Brooks, S. (2001). Working with animals in a healing context. *Reaching Today's Youth*, Winter, 19–22.

Brunner, J. (2004). Life as narrative. *Social Research, 71*, 691–711.

Burke, K. (1941). Four master tropes. *The Kenyon Review, 3*(4), 421–438.

Buttelmann, D., & Römpke, A. K. (2014). Anxiety-reducing effect: Dog, fish and plant in direct comparison. *Anthrozoös, 27*(2), 267–277.

Canadian Agency for Drugs and Technologies in Health (CADTH). (2012). Therapy dogs and horses for mental health: A review of the clinical effectiveness. Retrieved from CADTH https://www.cadth.ca/therapy-dogs-and-horses-mental-health-review-clinical-effectiveness.

Carter, B., & Charles, N. (2013). Animals, agency and resistance. *Journal for the Theory of Social Behaviour, 43*(3), 322–340.

Chandler, C. K. (2017). *Animal assisted therapy in counseling* (3rd ed.). New York: Routledge.

Chandler, C. K. (2018). Human-animal relational theory: A guide for animal-assisted counseling. *Journal of Creativity in Mental Health, 13*(4), 429–444.

Chandler, C., Portrie-Bethke, T., Minton, C., Fernando, D., & O'Callaghan, D. (2010). Matching animal-assisted therapy techniques and intentions with counseling guiding theories. *Journal of Mental Health Counseling, 32*(4), 354–374.

Corson, S. A., & O'Leary Corson, E. (1980). *Ethology and nonverbal communication in mental health: An interdisciplinary biopsychosocial exploration.* Pergamon Press.

Equine Assisted Growth and Learning Association. (2015). *Fundamentals of the EAGALA model: Practice untraining manual* (8th ed.). Santaquin, UT: EAGALA.

Fournier, A. K. (2016). PenPals: An examination of human-animal interaction as an outlet for healthy masculinity in prison. In C. Blazina & L. Kogan (Eds.), *Men and their dogs: A new understanding of man's best friend.* AG Switzerland: Springer.

Fournier, A. K., Geller, E. S., & Fortney, E. E. (2007). Human-animal interaction in a prison setting: Impact on criminal behavior, treatment progress, and social skills. *Behavior and Social Issues, 16*(1), 89–105. https://doi.org/10.5210/bsi.v16i1.385.

Fournier, A., Letson, E., Berry, T., & Pasiuk, E. (2018). Human-animal interaction and metaphor in equine-assisted psychotherapy: Empirical support for the EAGALA model. *Human-Animal Interaction Bulletin, 6*(1), 47–63.

Garrity, T. F., & Stallones, L. (1998). Effects of pet contact on human well-being: Review of recent research. In C. C. Wilson & D. C. Turner (Eds.), *Companion animals in human health* (pp. 3–22). Thousand Oaks, CA: Sage.

Gilbert, R. (2013). *Equine assisted psychotherapy: Provider perspectives and beliefs.* Doctoral dissertation. Available from ProQuest Dissertation and Theses database (UMI No. 3599176).

Havey, J., Vlasses, F. R., Vlasses, P. H., Ludwig-Beymer, P., & Hackbarth, D. (2014). The effect of animal-assisted therapy on pain medication use after joint replacement. *Anthrozoös, 27*(3), 361–369.

International Institute for Animal Assisted Play Therapy. (2018). *Certification manual; Animal assisted play therapy.* International Institute for Animal Assisted Play Therapy. Retrieved from http://risevanfleet.com/international/wp-content/uploads/2018/02/AAPT.CERTIFICATION.MANUAL.pdf.

Irvine, L. (2008). *If you tame me: Understanding our connection with animals.* Temple University Press.

Jerolmack, C. (2005). Our animals, our selves? Chipping away the human–animal divide. *Sociological Forum, 20*(4), 651–660. Springer Netherlands.

Karol, J. (2007). Applying a traditional individual psychotherapy model to equine-facilitated psychotherapy (EFP): Theory and method. *Clinical Child Psychology and Psychiatry, 12*(1), 77–90.

Kruger, K. A., & Serpell, J. A. (2006). Animal-assisted interventions in mental health: Definitions and theoretical foundations. In*Handbook on animal-assisted therapy: Foundations and guidelines for animal-assisted interventions* (pp. 33–48). Academic Press.

Kupers, T. (2001). Psychotherapy with men in prison. In G. Brooks & G. Good (Eds.), *A new handbook of counseling and psychotherapy approaches for men: A comprehensive guide to setting, problems, and treatment approaches* (pp. 170–184). San Francisco: Jossey-Bass.

Letson, E. A. (2012). *Metaphor: A key ingredient in equine-assisted psychotherapy and learning?* Unpublished master's thesis. Bemidji State University, Bemidji, MN.

Letson, E. A., & Fournier, A. K. (2017). The metaphor record. Createspace.com.

Lujan, K. (2012). *The challenges and discoveries in using equine assisted psychotherapy approaches by counseling practitioners in the southwest.* Dissertation, University of New Mexico.

Marino, L., & Colvin, C. M. (2015). Thinking Pigs. *International Journal of Comparative Psychology*, 28.

Merriam-Webster. (2019a). Agent. Retrieved from https://www.merriamebster.com/dictionary/agent.

Merriam-Webster. (2019b). Agency. Retrieved from https://www.merriamwebster.com/dictionary/agency.

Mueller, M. K., Fine, A. H., & O'Haire, M. E. (2019). Understanding the role of human-animal interaction in the family context. In A. H. Fine (Ed.), *Handbook on animal-assisted therapy: Foundations and guidelines for animal-assisted interventions* (5th ed.). San Diego, CA: Elsevier.

Myers, O. G. (1998). *Children and animals: Social development and our connections to other species.* Westview Press.

Nagasawa, M., Mitsui, S., En, S., Ohtani, N., Ohta, M., Sakuma, Y., et al. (2015). Oxytocin-gaze positive loop and the coevolution of human-dog bonds. *Science, 348*(6232), 333–336. https://doi.org/10.1126/science.1261022.

Notgrass, C. G., & Pettinelli, J. D. (2015). Equine-assisted psychotherapy: The equine-assisted growth and learning Association's model overview of equine-based modalities. *The Journal of Experimental Education, 38*(2), 162–174.

O'Callaghan, D. M. (2008). *Exploratory study of animal assisted therapy interventions used by mental health professionals.* Doctoral dissertation, University of North Texas.

Odendaal, J. S. (2000). Animal-assisted therapy—Magic or medicine? *Journal of Psychosomatic Research, 49*(4), 275–280. https://doi.org/10.1016/S0022-3999(00)00183-5.

Odendaal, J. S., & Meintjes, R. A. (2003). Neurophysiological correlates of affiliative behaviour between humans and dogs. *The Veterinary Journal, 165*(3), 296–301.

Phillips, J. (2001). Cultural construction of manhood in prison. *Psychology of Men & Masculinity, 2*(1), 13–23.

Quatman, T. (2015). *Essential psychodynamic psychotherapy: An acquired art.* Routledge.

Rogers, C. R. (1979). The foundations of the person-centered approach. *Education, 100*, 2.

Schultz, P. N., Remick-Barlow, G. A., & Robbins, L. (2007). Equine-assisted psychotherapy: A mental health promotion/intervention modality for children who have experienced intra-family violence. *Health and Social Care in the Community, 15*(3), 265–271.

Serpell, J. (1996). *In the company of animals: A study of human-animal relationships.* Cambridge University Press.

Serpell, J., McCune, S., Gee, N., & Griffin, J. A. (2017). Current challenges to research on animal-assisted interventions. *Applied Developmental Science, 21*(3), 223–233. https://doi.org/10.1080/10888691.2016.1262775.

Shaw, D. G. (2013). The torturer's horse: Agency and animals in history. *History and Theory, 52*(4), 146–167.

Sori, C. F., & Hughes, J. C. (2014). Animal-assisted play therapy: An interview with rise VanFleet. *The Family Journal, 22*(3), 350–356.

Thomas, L., & Lytle, M. (2016). *Transforming therapy through horses: Case stories teaching the Eagala model in action.* Santaquin, UT: Eagala.

VanFleet, R., & Faa-Thompson, T. (2017). *Animal assisted play therapy.* Professional Resource Press.

Velde, B. P., Cipriani, J., & Fisher, G. (2005). Resident and therapist views of animal-assisted therapy: Implications for occupational therapy practice. *Australian Occupational Therapy Journal, 52*(1), 43–50.

Vidrine, M., Owen-Smith, P., & Faulkner, P. (2002). Equine-facilitated group psychotherapy: Applications for therapeutic vaulting. *Issues in Mental Health Nursing, 23*(6), 587–603.

Wells, E. S., Rosen, L. W., & Walshaw, S. (1997). Use of feral cats in psychotherapy. *Anthrozoös, 10*(2–3), 125–130. https://doi.org/10.2752/089279397787001085.

Wilson, E. O. (1984). *Biophilia.* Cambridge, MA: Harvard University Press.

Yap, E., Scheinberg, A., & Williams, K. (2017). Attitudes to and beliefs about animal assisted therapy for children with disabilities. *Complementary Therapies in Clinical Practice, 26*, 47–52.

CHAPTER 6

Studying Animal-Assisted Intervention Through Citizen Science

Abstract Human–animal interaction (HAI) is an interface between two complex organisms; variables specific to the human (e.g., biology, learning history, personality), the animal (e.g., species, breed, biology, learning history, personality), and the situation (e.g., setting, length of interaction, treatment goals) impact how the human and animal interact and potential outcomes of the interaction. In addition to laboratory experiments testing basic phenomena, large-scale data collection is needed to parse out information on each variable as it relates to animal-assisted intervention (AAI). The citizen-science approach, which involves the public participating in the scientific process, could be useful in such an endeavor. Beyond individual studies addressing one variable at a time, the citizen-science approach could be used to grow large databases of many variables relevant to AAI. This chapter provides an example of the citizen-science approach applied to AAI. The study demonstrates the potential to gather data from a pool of nonscientists, capitalizing on the growing number of people and pets providing animal-assisted services.

Keywords Citizen Science • Animal-assisted intervention • Pet Partners • Factor analysis

Throughout this book, I have shared studies conducted with students and colleagues in the Human–Animal Interaction Laboratory. My intention in sharing these studies is to provide examples of how data can be gathered

A. K. Fournier, *Animal-Assisted Intervention*,
https://doi.org/10.1007/978-3-030-32972-3_6

and the kinds of questions practitioners and researchers can ask about animal-assisted intervention (AAI). At the risk of being repetitive, I will mention again that while helpful as examples, the findings are not conclusive. It is difficult to infer about the general population from small, homogeneous samples. In addition, the studies reviewed thus far have examined just a few of the variables related to AAI process and outcome. To really understand AAI, we need much more data—data on many more animals, practitioners, clients, situations, and settings. In essence, the field would benefit from large-scale data collection, beyond the limitations of one study with one sample. One way to gather large-scale data is to partner with citizens in empirical endeavors.

Citizen Science

Citizen science is the involvement of the public in scientific research (Citizen-Science Association 2019). Although the term had not yet been coined, citizen science dates back to at least the 1830s. In 1837, William Whewell received the Royal Medal for his research on ocean tides. He learned about ocean tides at beaches and harbors worldwide through reports of thousands of volunteers who recorded tidal information in their part of the world. The project included volunteers measuring tides at over 650 tidal stations at exactly the same time, around the clock, for two weeks. This mass of data was necessary to better understand the ocean tides around the world and was possible because thousands of citizens volunteered to contribute to the scientific process by gathering data for the project (Cooper 2016).

Today, there are thousands of citizen science projects supported by millions of volunteers around the world. A relatively recent increase in this approach is attributed to communication technology, appreciation for the public as a free and available resource, and granting agencies encouraging or requiring science outreach (Silvertown 2009). Projects are largely in the natural sciences—biology, environmental science, geography—and can range in the level of citizen participation. Bonney and colleagues categorize citizen science projects into one of three categories: contributory, collaborative, or co-created (2009). These categories involve citizens passively contributing data, gathering and analyzing data, or helping with all levels of the project including development, respectively. In another framework, Haklay (2013) distinguishes between four levels of participation in citizen science. The most basic is level 1—crowdsourcing—in which citizens act as sensors, merely going about their world while carrying sensors to measure variables and report back to the researcher. Level 4—extreme citizen science—is collaborative, wherein citizens contribute to defining the research problem, in addition to collecting and analyzing the data. The framework was developed with geographical research in mind, but could apply to other disciplines, including those in the anthrozoology field.

Citizen Science in Anthrozoology

Although the field of anthrozoology is quite broad, citizen-science projects within the field have had a narrower focus, typically recording animal behavior patterns (e.g., identifying monarch butterfly migration patterns, describing bee habitats). Although citizen-science research has not yet addressed HAI per se, studies on animal behavior certainly inform and impact interactions between humans and animals. For example, a "cat tracker" study in Australia involved pet owners tracking their pet cats with a GPS collar to explore their movement (Roetman et al. 2018). The findings changed pet cat management such that after seeing results a substantial proportion of cat owners reported containing their cat more than before (e.g., keeping the cat indoors at night). There are a growing number of projects within canine science, in which dog owners provide researchers with information on their canine companions. In some studies citizens contribute by bringing their dogs to a laboratory for a lab-based experiment (e.g., Bensky et al. 2013). Other projects are questionnaire-based; citizens report on their dog's behavior through surveys (e.g., Fratkin and Baker 2013). Regarding other domesticated animals, Krueger et al. (2019) conducted a crowdsourcing study on equine behavior; the researchers were studying horses that open doors and gates. Such behaviors are entertaining (e.g., The Telegraph 2013) but can be dangerous for both humans and animals. Citizen science can be useful in studying infrequent behavior such as this, since it would take a much longer time to acquire an adequate sample size using traditional research methods. Beyond behavior patterns, there are a growing number of studies looking at animal cognition.

Brian Hare is a cognitive psychologist who studies dog cognition. His research team uses citizen science to gather data on the cognitive abilities of dogs. Dog owners can register with a website (dognition.com), engage their dog in tasks, and provide information about their dog's performance. The owner receives feedback about their dog's abilities and preferences and the information they share about their dog becomes part of a large research database. The researchers use the data to answer empirical questions about canine cognition.

Citizen Science in Animal-Assisted Intervention

AAI is a growing field, with practitioners around the globe bringing an assortment of animals into various settings for the benefit of human health and well-being. The number of animals and handlers involved in AAI is extensive, but difficult to estimate as there is no overarching organization charged with accreditation, regulation, or documentation of services. Instead, AAI prevalence can be estimated from the organizations that certify therapy animals and/or their handlers. For example, the Equine-Assisted Growth and Learning Association (Eagala), which trains and certifies practitioners in equine-assisted intervention, reports 60,000 clients were served by its members in 2018 (Eagala 2019). Pet Partners, an organization that registers animal-handler teams, reports 3 million animal visits are provided annually by their members (Pet Partners 2019).

Despite the large number of AAI services being provided, we know very little about the interactions that happen between the humans and animals during these interventions.

Chubak and Hawkes (2016) studied safety-related practices for animal-assisted activity (AAA) programs in oncology hospitals. They surveyed top pediatric oncology hospitals to learn more about AAA for hospitalized children with cancer. They found that most AAA programs involved dogs, and that human–animal interaction (HAI) occurred in waiting rooms and individual patient rooms. Results indicated some similarities in practice (e.g., most require handwashing after an animal visit), but also found significant variation between hospitals (e.g., some hospitals require visits be supervised by a hospital staff member while others do not). The researchers conclude there is at least some variation in AAA practice and no data to date on which practices are safe or effective.

Our team conducted a study to gather data on exactly which kinds of behavioral interactions occur during AAA and whether certain interactions are more or less potent for human health outcomes. The paradigm is consistent with citizen science in that citizens, not researchers, were gathering data. It is worth sharing here, as this general paradigm could be useful on a larger scale to (1) take advantage of the abundant practitioners impassioned about their work and (2) create large databases on the multitude of variables in AAI.

Citizen Science with Pet Partners

Founded in 1977 (formerly known as Delta Society), Pet Partners is a national nonprofit organization registering handlers as volunteer teams providing "animal-assisted interactions" (Pet Partners 2019). The organization trains handlers of multiple species (e.g., dog, cat, horse, bird). The organization supports and evaluates human–animal teams for visiting animal programs in various settings (e.g., hospitals, nursing homes, schools). Animal-assisted interactions may include animal-assisted therapy, education, or activity. Pet Partners generously collaborated with our research team to conduct a study wherein we gathered HAI data through the citizen-science approach. Animal handlers conducted their AAI work as usual and recorded data on individual sessions.

Practitioner Participation

A total of 100 adults agreed to participate. The sample comprised mostly women (81.8%, $n = 81$), with 18.2% men ($n = 19$). All participants were involved with Pet Partners and volunteered their time to bring their animal for animal-assisted interactions. Practitioner participant age ranged from 15 to 86 years old ($M = 56.02$, $SD = 13.95$); the median age was 58 and the mode was 71. Approximately 80% of participants were above age 46, making most participants middle-aged or older. Regarding race or ethnicity, 1% ($n = 1$) of participants identified as American Indian, 3% ($n = 3$) identified as Asian, 3% ($n = 3$) identified as Latinx, and 92.9% ($n = 92$) identified as White.

Materials included a background questionnaire, session log, and the Human–Animal Interaction Scale (HAIS). The background questionnaire was created for this study, asking basic demographic questions about the participant and their therapy animal(s), as well as information about their AAI training and experience. The session log was also created for this study, designed to record session logistics (e.g., setting, date, time) and a brief description of the session. The 24-item HAIS was embedded within the session log so that practitioners could report on the behavioral HAI that occurred during the session. All data gathered pertained to the setting and the animal; no information was gathered from the AAI recipient (i.e., patient, client). Instead, participants reported on their animal—were they *petted* or *talked to*, did they *sniff* and *lick* the intervention recipient? This allowed us to gather data on the session without infringing on the recipient's privacy or relying on sensitive data to be gathered by volunteers who were not trained in research methodology and ethics.

Participants were recruited through an email sent from Pet Partners, describing the study and inviting them to a free webinar to learn more. Those who attended the webinar were given (1) a link to complete informed consent online, followed by (2) a link to complete the background questionnaire online, and (3) a link to the online session log, which they could complete once per session for an unlimited number of sessions. Because AAI occurs in a variety of settings, we asked participants to complete at least three session logs within each setting they typically visited. Participants were instructed to go about their work as they normally would. The research was not meant to impact session setting, duration, frequency, etc. The animal handler conducted a Pet Partners session as usual; once the session was over, they completed the session log. The logs were completed through an online survey platform, so participants could complete them on a mobile device immediately after the session for best recall.

Animal-Handler Team Demographics

When asked about workload, handlers reported a wide range of session frequencies. AAI work ranged from 1 to 6 days per week (M = 1.81, SD = 1.24). Regarding individual sessions, participants reported conducting 1 to 100 sessions per week (M = 12.49, SD = 13.28). Animals were of several species. A proportion of the participants (n = 23) reported working with more than one intervention animal. Thus, the 100 respondents reported on a total of 126 animals of several species. Dogs made up most of the sample (87.3%, n = 110), followed by cats (n = 8, 6.3%), rabbits (n = 6, 4.8%), a horse (n = 1, 0.8%), and a rat (n = 1, 0.8%). For the dogs, there were a range of breeds, from chihuahua to bull mastiff. Golden retriever and Labrador retriever were the most common (n = 21 and 17 respectively). Therapy animal age ranged from 1 to 13 years (M = 6.20, SD = 2.98).

Participants were asked to complete multiple session logs, at least three from each setting in which they provided AAI. This resulted in 746 session logs completed over a six-month research period. For the majority of these sessions, the therapy animal was a dog and the session was described as AAA in the form of an unstructured visit. The remainder of the findings are reported on just these sessions (83.6%, n = 624).

The number of individual session logs completed by specific Pet Partners handlers ranged from 3 to 91. Data provide information on the nature of the session (i.e., type, location, length) and the behavioral interactions that occurred during the session. Pet Partners workload and session logistics were highly variable. The sessions ranged from 1 minute to 6 hours and 30 minutes, with a mean duration of 39.2 minutes. This is consistent with Glenk's review of canine-assisted intervention research which showed dogs working from 1 to 6 hours at a time (2017). The most common session length was 1 hour, making up 14.2% of the sessions. Sessions took place in a variety of settings, with the most common being hospitals (60.6%) and nursing homes (55.6%). Within these settings, animal handlers reported positive outcomes for clients/patients, families, and staff.

Respondents were asked to report the lag time between the end of the Pet Partners session and completion of the session log. Responses varied; 23.2% (n = 145) were completed within the hour following the session, 26.0% (n = 162) were completed 1 to 4 hours after, 14.6% (n = 91) were completed 4–8 hours later, and 17.8% (n = 111) were completed 8–24 hours later. A smaller proportion was completed 1–2 days later (6.9%, n = 43), 2–5 days later (5.4%, n = 34), and more than 5 days later (6.1%, n = 38).

Human–Animal Interaction Analysis

The HAIS was embedded in the session log. Respondents reported interactions from the animal's perspective, recording interactions toward the animal (e.g., the animal was *petted*) and from the animal (e.g., the animal *sniffed* the human). Figure 6.1 shows the ratings for behaviors emitted from the human toward the animal during sessions, limited to sessions in hospitals (n = 295), nursing homes (n = 111), and schools (n = 24). Across the sample, each of the behaviors was endorsed, with some more common than others. From the graph, you can see the most common behaviors toward the animal were *watch*, *spend time near*, and *pet*. Separated by setting, it is clear there were similarities and differences across the locations.

Although this research was descriptive and did not investigate reasons for differences between settings, we can speculate possibilities. For example, *talking to*, *kissing*, and *playing* with the animal were rated higher in nursing homes than in hospitals. This could be because of the Pet Partners teams that visited each setting (e.g., perhaps handlers with dogs that like to play go to nursing homes more than hospitals), behaviors that were allowed per institutional policy (e.g., playing is allowed in nursing homes

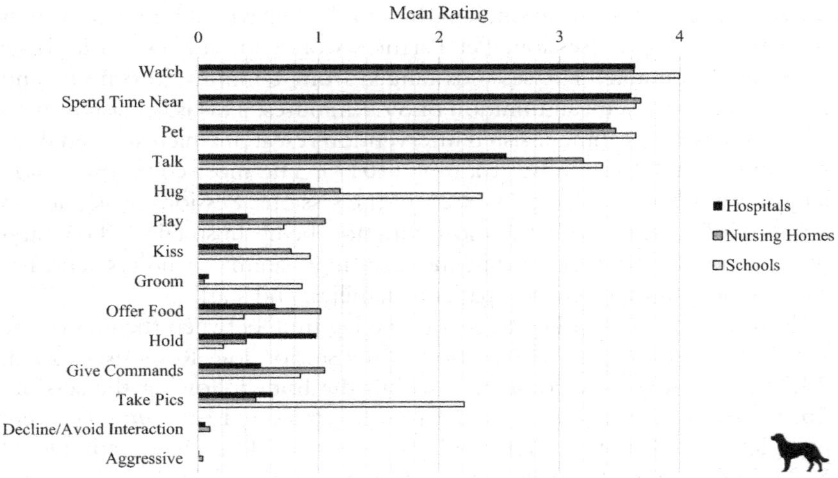

Fig. 6.1 Human-initiated HAI during Pet Partners sessions. Graph showing interactions from clients/patients toward therapy dogs in Pet Partners sessions. Data reflect sessions that occurred in hospitals ($n = 295$), nursing homes ($n = 111$), and schools ($n = 24$)

more than hospitals), or for some other reason. Note that *taking pictures* was rated much higher in school settings than in hospitals or nursing homes. We can imagine intervention recipients at schools, including middle school, high school, and college settings, would have greater access to mobile phones and be more likely to take pictures than nursing home residents. We should consider factors such as these when examining HAI within an AAI. Observing or reporting a behavior during a specific intervention does not mean that behavior will reliably occur in other, similar situations. There could be factors specific to that intervention, animal, client, or setting that elicited the behavior.

Figure 6.2 shows data on the animal-initiated behavior during the sessions. Similar to human-initiated behavior, there were a variety of behaviors reported and some were rated higher than others. *Initiating interaction* and *obeying commands* were rated the highest. Note that the list of animal behaviors includes four items addressing negative or undesirable behaviors from the animal: *decline/avoid interaction*, *make unfriendly sounds*, *make a mess/inconvenience*, and *aggressive behavior*. Mean ratings for *decline/avoid interaction* and *make unfriendly sounds* were quite low

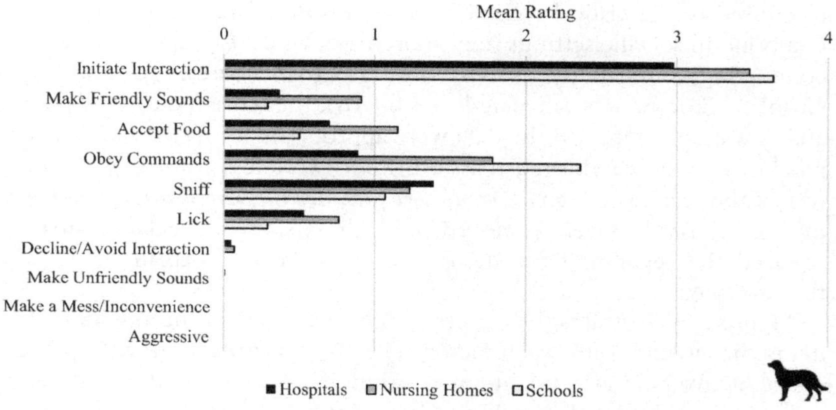

Fig. 6.2 Animal-initiated HAI during Pet Partners sessions. Graph showing behaviors emitted by the therapy dog in Pet Partners sessions that occurred in hospitals (n = 295), nursing homes (n = 111), and schools (n = 24)

relative to the more positive, desirable behaviors. *Make a mess/inconvenience* and *aggressive behavior* did not occur at all, according to the animal handlers. Similar to behaviors emitted by the client, behaviors emitted by the therapy animal differed by setting. For example, *obeying commands* was most common in school settings and *making friendly sounds* was most common in nursing homes. Again, we cannot say these patterns will be found across all sessions. Rather, it is important to study AAI in this way to determine whether there is a "typical" interaction occurring in certain settings, with certain animals, or with certain clients/patients. All of this information could be helpful in developing the most effective and efficient AAIs. In that regard, we can further analyze these data to detect interaction patterns that inform AAI practices.

Factor Analysis of Behavioral Interactions

Exploratory factor analysis was conducted to determine whether scores on individual behaviors clustered together into larger behavior groups or factors. This can tell us whether individual behaviors grouped together to represent larger, unobserved constructs. Conducting factor analysis like this can be useful in development of psychological instruments and theory (e.g., Coleman et al. 2016). Within the field of anthrozoology, researchers have used this statistical technique to better understand the human–animal bond in specific settings (e.g., Porcher et al. 2004). The first step was conducting a reliability analysis on the HAIS scores. To do this, a Cronbach's alpha was calculated ($\alpha = 0.818$); the score indicated that reliability was adequate and the data were appropriate for factor analysis. The reliability analysis indicated that four items were less consistent with the rest of the scale: the items *groom*, *take pics*, *decline/avoid interaction*, and *aggressive behavior* were removed from the analysis. The factor analysis reduced the remaining ten items into three factors, explaining 72% of the variance.

Figure 6.3 illustrates the results of the analysis, showing the individual items that loaded onto each factor. The three factors seem to represent casual, active, and affectionate interaction. The factors are listed in order of largest to smallest eigenvalues. *Casual* interaction explained the largest proportion of the variance, then *active*, then *affectionate*. Factor 1—casual interaction—included *watch*, *spend time near*, *pet*, and *talk*. At face value, these behaviors could perhaps represent an underlying construct of casual behaviors; each of these behaviors could be performed with an animal that you know well, such as a pet, but also an animal that you have just met. Factor 2 included the items *give commands*, *offer food*, and *play*. These

Fig. 6.3 Three-factor model of human-initiated HAI. Figure illustrating the three factors identified through factor analysis of Pet Partners session logs ($n = 624$). Items on the HAIS clustered into three categories reflecting casual, active, and affectionate behavior

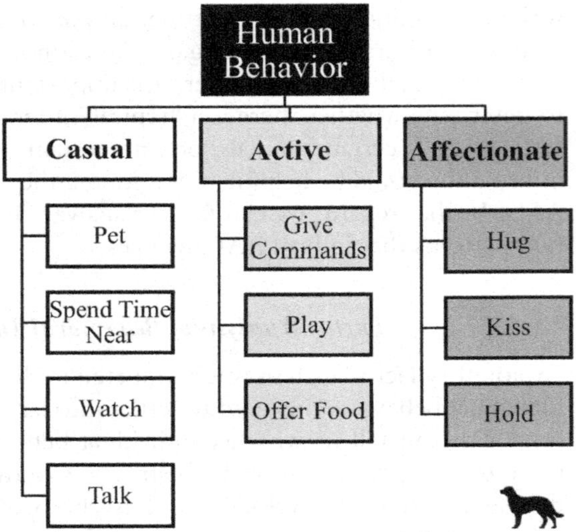

behaviors are more physically active and often occur together; perhaps that is why they clustered together. The third factor included items that involve more intimate, affectionate contact—*hug*, *kiss*, and *hold*. These are behaviors that require close physical contact and you could say require or represent a more intimate or intense interaction. Within the factors, items are listed from the largest factor loading to the smallest; the top item listed explained the greatest variance, then the next item, and so on. *Pet* was the item that explained the greatest variance within the casual behaviors, *give commands* was greatest for active behaviors, and *hug* was greatest for affectionate behaviors.

Note that although these factors emerged in this dataset, they may not emerge in other samples; one study cannot determine whether this is a reliable finding. Instead, we can replicate this study with other samples and see if we find the same thing. Only then can we be confident that individual behaviors (e.g., *hugging*, *kissing*, or *holding* an animal) are part of a larger construct (e.g., affectionate interaction) and test its properties. For example, if this three-factor model were to be confirmed, I would be curious to know whether the different types of behaviors—casual, active, and affectionate—result in differential outcomes. Do *affectionate* behaviors result in a greater anodyne effect than *active* behaviors? Is *casual* interaction associated with stress for the therapy animal more or less than *affectionate* interaction? Are interaction–outcome relationships related to other factors, like animal species, breed, or learning history? These are just a few examples of the kinds of questions we can ask to dig deeper into specific interactions and associated outcomes.

Role of the Therapy Animal

Participants were asked the open-ended question "how do you think your animal helped the clients/patients?" Written responses ($n = 620$) were analyzed for themes, following the constant comparative method (Brunner 2004) described earlier, then coded by two independent researchers. Interrater reliability for coding was determined by calculating Cohen's kappa statistic; kappa = 0.325, $p < 0.001$; and suggested good reliability (Altman 1991). In 1.1% of the logs ($n = 7$), the animal handler reported that the animal didn't seem to help or they couldn't tell how the animal may have helped. For 17.9% of the logs ($n = 111$), the content was either a concrete description of the session (e.g., "Banjo visited a child with leukemia") or a statement on how much the client enjoyed or appreciated the

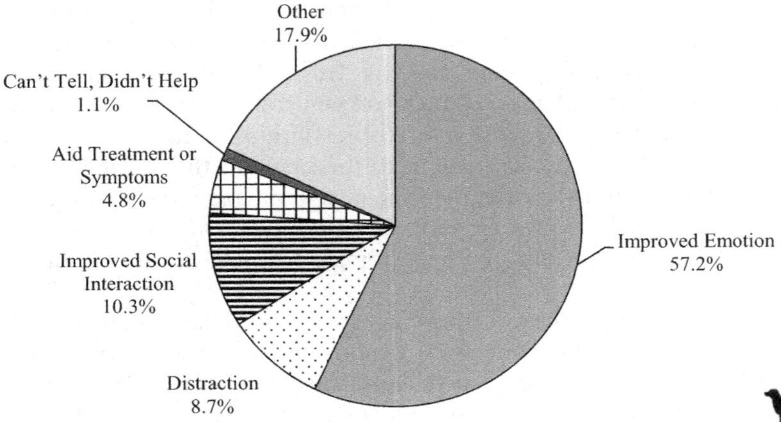

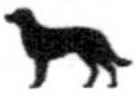

Fig. 6.4 Practitioner perception of the animal's role in animal-assisted activity. Pet Partners practitioners reported their perception of the dog's role in assisting during sessions. Comments resulted in four themes. Helping to improve emotion was the most common role reported

visit (e.g., "they were very thankful"). These statements were categorized as Other, as they indicated a positive response but did not fit a category on *how* the animal may have helped the individuals involved. The remaining logs (n = 502) included a description of how the handler perceived the animal to have helped the intervention recipient(s). A total of four themes emerged from these responses, illustrated in Fig. 6.4.

Of the 502 session logs in which the animal's role was described, improved emotion was the most frequently reported at 57.2% (n = 354). In these sessions, participants reported their animal helped someone feel joy, happiness, calm, less anxious or fearful, and less stressed. Next, a proportion of participants suggested their animal helped by improving social interaction (10.3%, n = 64). In this category, handlers indicated their animal got the person engaged with them or other people in the room; they also described people as being more expressive, verbally and nonverbally. Distraction was a third theme, indicated in 8.7% of cases (n = 54). These responses were given largely in treatment settings (e.g., hospitals, clinics); respondents indicated the animal helped intervention recipients forget their troubles or forget where they were for a little while. Finally, 4.8% felt their therapy animal helped intervention recipients by aiding treatment or symptoms (n = 30). This took the form of reduced physical pain or psychological symptoms.

One could argue that animal handlers describing the benefits of their pets in an intervention they facilitated are inherently biased. For example, don't we all think our pets are important and helpful? Can we rely on the reports of handlers? These are good points and we cannot be certain that these findings accurately reflect the role of the therapy animals in the sessions. Further research is necessary, preferably using multiple methods. Interviews with the intervention recipients themselves would be helpful to confirm or deny the speculation of the animal handlers. Until then, we can compare the present findings with previous research to determine whether it is consistent with other reports. In that case, a study by Shen et al. (2018) conducted a systematic review of qualitative research on AAI, exploring the mechanism of effectiveness in seven studies. They identified six themes on how animals assist in interventions; distraction, improved emotion, and increased behavioral activation (e.g., social interaction) were among the mechanisms identified.

Within the various settings, animal handlers reported what might be described as a ripple effect, where animal visits affect humans beyond the specific target. For example, when describing reading programs, there were descriptions of smiles and cheers from the children, but also the librarians and adult library patrons. When dogs visited hospitals, handlers reported they also impacted patient families, people in the waiting room, and medical staff on the floor. This is consistent with research on the benefits of dog visits for nontargeted staff (Barker et al. 2005; Ladd and Barker 2017).

HAI Across Animal Role

Statistical tests were conducted to determine whether the animal's role, as reported by animal handlers, was related to HAI. A one-way ANOVA was calculated, comparing total HAIS scores across the four themes. As Fig. 6.5 shows, there was a small but significant difference in HAI between themes. Specifically, sessions where aiding symptoms or treatment was the reported outcome involved greater amounts of reported HAI (M = 32.13, SD = 11.87) than when the outcome was improved emotion (M = 26.48, SD = 11.71), $F(3, 428) = 2.13$, $p = 0.023$. Please note there were similarities within reporters, such that some animal

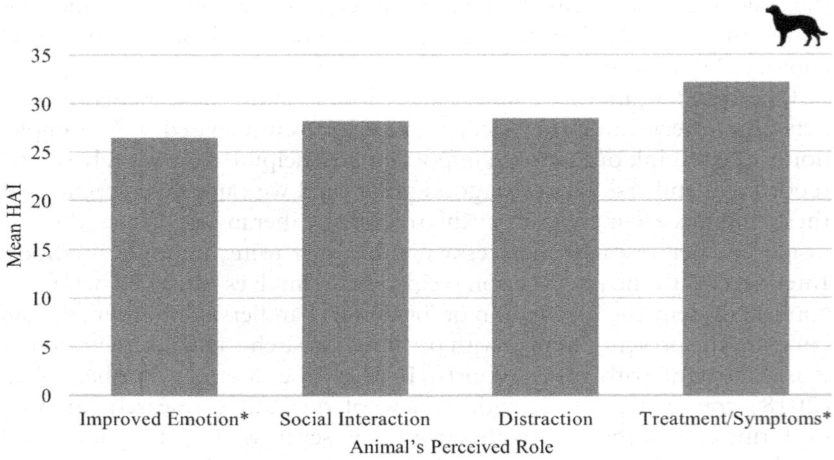

Fig. 6.5 Mean HAI across animal's perceived role. This graph shows the mean HAIS score across the four roles identified by Pet Partners practitioners. Behavioral HAI was greater in sessions where the animal helped with treatment/symptoms than sessions where the perceived role was to assist with improved mood. $^*p < 0.05$

handlers were more likely to report certain themes; there may also be patterns in their report on the HAIS. Because both variables are quite subjective, and these findings are confounded by animal handler, animal, and in some cases the setting, we cannot say from these data that these levels of HAI lead to specific outcomes. We can only say that the data in this sample show patterns in responding such that HAIS scores seem to be associated with perceived outcome themes. More analysis of these data is needed; research using experimental methods is necessary to draw cause-and-effect conclusions.

Discussion

In this study behavioral HAI data were gathered from AAI practitioners to (1) examine behavioral HAI occurring in AAA and (2) test the utility of citizen science for AAI research. Session logs indicated a range of interactive behaviors occurred during sessions, with differences across settings. Data such as this could be examined further to test for differences across therapy animals and practitioners. It stands to reason that one dog may do more sniffing and licking than another dog. Research on dog personality has identified behavioral differences between and *within* breed (e.g., Mirkó et al. 2012). Furthermore, some practitioners may provide treats for patients to feed their dog while others may not. These variations in interaction alter the experience and could have important effects for the intervention outcome. Differences should be examined in AAI program evaluation and tested more rigorously in research, with the goal of getting to a place where we can reliably predict outcomes from particular animals, interactions, or doses. In addition to providing a window into the interactions occurring during AAI, this research tested the citizen-science approach as a data collection method.

One mass email was sent to registered handlers. Of the 3000 people emailed, 100 completed the study. Although a response rate of 3% limits our ability to make inferences, the study demonstrates the potential to gather data on AAI from practitioners. Cumulatively, they completed over 700 session logs, reporting on session logistics and interactions that occurred between their animal and clients/patients. This volume of data was provided over a six-month period, prompted only by an email. There was no monetary reward; volunteers received a final report and certificate of participation. Although not systematically recorded, many participants added comments about their excitement for the project, acknowledged the need for evidence on AAI, and expressed their gratitude for the opportunity to contribute to the research base. Given the volume of practitioners providing these interventions, and their potential enthusiasm for contributing to research, citizen science could be an important tool for AAI research. There is also something special about practitioners like those who contributed to this study. Few other fields have thousands of volunteers providing services for physical or psychological health. Pet Partners has been contributing to AAI since 1977 and currently has more than 13,000 registered teams (Pet Partners 2019). Most of the animal handlers volunteer their time, often several hours a day, bringing their animals to various settings to reduce distress, provide a distraction, and bring people joy.

Limitations Specific to Citizen Science

In part, thinking empirically means thinking critically, ruling out alternative explanations and acknowledging limitations of research design, method, or findings. Any empirical investigation will have shortcomings, but citizen science brings unique limitations related to the sample and quality of the data. Hecht and Spicer Rice (2015) discuss the use of citizen science in canine behavior research. They list several data-quality challenges for citizen science relevant to our study, including sampling error and data quality.

Sampling Error

In each research project, we are curious about the population—we want to know how AAI impacts human health and well-being. But we cannot observe all AAI recipients, so we gather a sample of people. We study that sample and hope to infer findings on the sample to the population. Sampling error is the error caused by observing a sample instead of the whole population (Lynn 2004). The sample can never "look" exactly like the population, so there is always some level of sampling error. As researchers, we aim to reduce the degree of sampling error for each study. Sampling error can be estimated by examining the similarity of the sample to the population. The more similar the sample is to the population, the more confident we can be in generalizing the study's findings. Being involved in research is voluntary; people have the choice whether to participate. For the present study, sampling error is an issue on two levels: who chose to participate and which session they chose to report on.

First, we must wonder whether the Pet Partners practitioners who chose to participate are representative of all Pet Partners practitioners: are they, their therapy animal(s), and their AAI recipients like those in the whole population? As was mentioned earlier, the recruitment email was sent to over 3000 Pet Partners practitioners and 100 of them completed the study. We cannot be confident that what we found with 3% of the population is reflective of all AAI or even all Pet Partners AAI. Self-selection bias is error that occurs when respondents can decide entirely for themselves whether they want to participate in a study (Lavrakas 2008). Typically, citizen scientists self-select into the study; they are not randomly selected. In our study, there could be systematic differences between those who did and did not participate in the research, and those differences could impact the findings. For example, perhaps the practitioners who volunteered for the study tend to be more outgoing, in general, than those who declined. It is possible that a more outgoing practitioner behaves in such a way as to impact the AAI, affecting the way the therapy animal and patient/client interact. If that were the case, the data we have would be skewed to indicate a greater level of HAI than is actually occurring in the population. This is just one example of how one potential factor could impact the data. A stronger method would be to randomly select practitioners to participate in the study. Theoretically, a random sample would include practitioners with varying degrees of outgoingness, or any other relevant factors, relative to the population. Future studies could make efforts to randomly select practitioners to recruit as citizen scientists, rather than the convenience sample used here.

Data Quality

We should be concerned about the quality (i.e., accuracy) of any data we gather, whether for assessment of an individual client, evaluation of an AAI program, or empirical research. When research data are gathered by nonscientists, there are some specific factors to consider. In the present study, factors that may have impacted the accuracy of the data are recall, interpretation, and expectancy bias.

Recall is an issue whenever we ask someone to complete a self-report, wherein they are asked a question about a behavior or experience. The greater the time between the behavior and the report, the greater is the concern about accurate recall (i.e., do they remember accurately?). We don't know how accurately the practitioners recalled specific behaviors when completing the session logs. This is true when completing the log immediately following the session, and especially when completing it sometime later. For a proportion of the data, there was substantial lag time between the session and completion of the session log—up to several days later in some cases. This is an issue to consider in follow-up research.

There was also room for error in the practitioners' interpretation of HAI during the sessions. They were asked to complete the session log based on their observations, rating a behavior from 0, meaning it did not occur, to 4, meaning it happened a great deal. We don't know whether behaviors were rated consistently across practitioners. It was possible that one practitioner rated an interaction as a 2 while another rated the same interaction as a 3. The webinar provided information and examples of the rating scale, but there was no formal training as is suggested in behavioral research (Thornton and Zorich 1980). Bird et al. (2014) discuss error and bias in citizen science datasets and provide suggestions for addressing the limitations. Regarding error, researchers may be concerned about nonexpert volunteers' ability to gather precise, accurate data. This can sometimes be addressed by selecting presence-only-type dependent measures. It is easier, and thus there is less room for error, to record presence versus absence of something than it is to quantify something (Bird et al. 2014).

With regard to HAIS data, it would be easier for volunteers to indicate whether a behavior did or did not occur, compared with the rating format currently used. With the rating, there is room for error in recall, as well as interrater variability in ratings. Future research could use a revised version of the HAIS in which practitioners simply indicate whether each behavior occurred, rather than applying a number to represent the degree to which it occurred. However, error could also occur with regard to macro-identification of behaviors (e.g., some might interpret a sound emitted by an animal as friendly while others interpret it as unfriendly). Human–animal dynamics are defined and interpreted differently across cultures (Gray and Young 2011). Operational definitions were provided for each of the items on the HAIS, spelling out what it means to *pet*, *hug*, *hold*, and so on. The HAIS observer form in Appendix B provides those definitions. As you can see, there is still room for interpretation within the definitions and thus inconsistencies in recording the presence or absence of a behavior.

Expectancy bias occurs when the researcher's expectations about the results of the study cause them to behave in ways that elicit the behavior they expected. It can also cause the researcher to see what they expected to see, even if that observation is inaccurate (Shuller and McNamara 1976). Herzog (2011) discussed bias in the literature on pets and human well-being, making the point that researchers are at risk to make erroneous positive results when studying a topic in which they have a vested interest. Researchers drawn to study the human–animal bond may be pet lovers who have personal convictions about the power of animals, and these convictions can bias research methods and results. Gathering AAI data via the intervention animal handler is subject to the same, and perhaps greater, risk of erroneous conclusions.

We can imagine that the handlers may have had expectations about their animal and how they help people, shaping what they saw during sessions and subsequently what they recorded on the session logs. This could have impacted the individual behaviors recorded on the HAIS as well as the open-ended comments that resulted in themes on the animal's role in the intervention. While expectancies can be an issue in any research project, it is particularly important here, because the practitioners were reporting on their animal, their *pet*, or their *partner*. They reported on the demographic questionnaire, and through emails sent after the study, that they believe in the power of animals, including their own pet, helping people. This perception of their pet and the work could have impacted their report on the session logs. We don't know if they rated *hug* high because there was actually a lot of hugging happening or because they have seen their dog hugged in the past, they see their dog as the kind of dog that people hug, and they assumed or incorrectly recalled that hugging occurred. The HAIS brings in additional potential for expectancy bias. Having the list of behaviors to rate may suggest to the practitioners that these behaviors *should* occur and prompt them to recall behaviors that didn't *actually* occur. This could be an issue for anyone completing the HAIS and should be addressed when training practitioners or researchers.

Validation of Citizen-Science Data

These potential limitations—sampling bias and inaccurate data collection—are an issue with citizen science. Silvertown (2009) recommends that data gathered through citizen science be validated. As an example, the researchers on dognition.com conducted a study to determine the validity of their data (Stewart et al. 2015). You can imagine dog owners asked to report on their dog's cognitive abilities might be biased in favor of their pet. Who wants to tell a researcher that their dog can't do suggested tasks? In addition to expectancy bias, the dognition data are subject to limited accuracy because of differences in operational definitions, just like the present study. To validate their data, Stewart and colleagues compared reports from citizen scientists who contributed data through the website with conventional lab-based studies using similar data. The citizen-science data replicated laboratory data and there was little if any evidence of fabrication by the citizen volunteers (Stewart et al. 2015). Consistent with this practice, Fig. 6.6 shows HAIS data from the Pet Partners study with a laboratory study in which the same session was recorded by students participating in the session and researchers observing the session. Thus, the figure shows a comparison of HAIS items reported by (a) Pet Partners observing an intervention, (b) students participating in a laboratory-based intervention, and (c) researchers observing the same laboratory-based intervention.

The data are graphed on a line graph for easier comparison. The three-factor model identified in the factor analysis has been integrated, so that interactive behaviors are listed in the order of the three factors—casual, active, and affectionate behaviors. As you can see, the general shape of the three lines is similar. Pet Partners data did not vary much from the

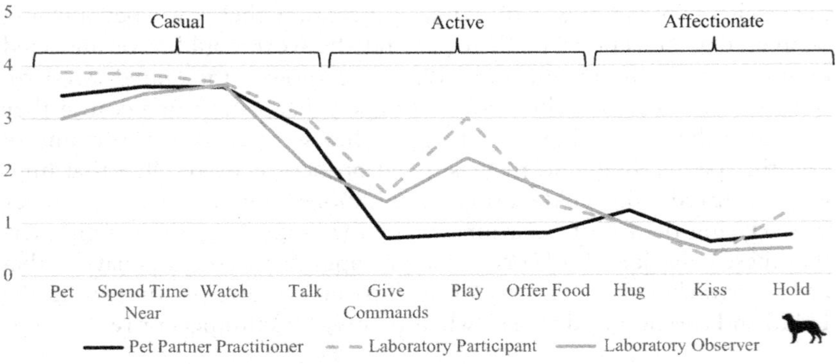

Fig. 6.6 Comparison of HAI reports by practitioners, participants, and observers. To help validate citizen-science data, HAI reports by Pet Partners practitioners are compared to that of laboratory participants and observers. Reports are similar for individual items as well as categories in the three-factor model

laboratory-based intervention data. The biggest difference seems to be within the active factor, on the item *play*. This item was rated lower in the Pet Partners study than in the laboratory study. This discrepancy could be because of a number of variables, only one of which is a reflection of a shortcoming of the Pet Partners reports (e.g., error in recall, bias). Other potential explanations are a real difference between HAI in basic versus applied settings, differences in interactive behavior of the different animals or human recipients, factors within the different settings, and other unknown variables. Since the Pet Partners data were largely gathered in hospitals and nursing homes, it could be that play was not a behavior allowed or possible for the patients in those settings. Perhaps there was no space or it was not safe for patients to be playing with a dog.

Beyond *play*, the shape of the curves created by the lines is remarkably similar. For all three respondent types, casual behaviors were rated the highest, then active, then affectionate. In laboratory studies, we have repeatedly found research ***participants*** rate HAIS items higher than ***researchers*** making observations of the same intervention session. Similarly, the Pet Partners data were more like those of the laboratory observers than the laboratory participants. The similarity of the scores across these three types of respondents is also important in addressing whether Pet Partners practitioners were biased in reporting on their animals' interactions with intervention recipients.

Regarding HAIS scores, bias could be reflected in higher ratings on positive, desirable behaviors and lower ratings on negative, undesirable behaviors. Regarding the latter, *decline/avoid interaction* and *aggressive behavior* were rated similarly (i.e., relatively low) across all three respondent types. Furthermore, Pet Partners rated *decline/avoid interaction* ($M = 0.074$) more similarly to laboratory observers ($M = 0.071$) than to laboratory participants ($M = 0.040$). The same was true for *aggressive behavior*—Pet Partners ratings ($M = 0.010$) were more like those of laboratory observers ($M = 0.000$) than like those of participants ($M = 0.040$). Although not definitive, these data suggest that biased responses by the citizen scientists had little effect if any on the results.

Conclusion

This chapter introduced citizen science and demonstrated its use in studying AAI. The Pet Partners study showed gathering data via AAI practitioners is possible and may be a useful tool in creating large-scale databases needed to explore the many variables relevant to AAI process and outcome. Despite the utility of the citizen-science approach, the number of published research articles is still limited. Burgess and colleagues studied the lack of citizen-science publications in the area of biodiversity (Burgess et al. 2017). Their survey of biodiversity scientists and citizen-science project managers identified several barriers, including low awareness or bias among scientists and inconsistencies in data quality.

Although citizen science is a relatively new method in anthrozoology, the practice has been utilized by researchers in other fields for quite some time. Literature on citizen science in the natural sciences can be useful in applying the method for animal-assisted work. Silvertown (2009) provides guidelines for good citizen-science practice: (a) publicly collected data should be validated, (b) data collection methods should be well designed and standardized, (c) any assumptions should be explicit, (d) research should be hypothesis-driven, and (e) citizen scientists should receive feedback on their contribution. The Pet Partners study met several of these recommendations. Comparisons with previous studies suggest the practitioners recorded observations similar to trained researchers, an important initial validation of the data quality. We used a standardized data collection method—the HAIS—and provided feedback on the citizen scientists contribution via a final report. Given the exploratory nature of the study, and the lack of empirical information on behavioral HAI in AAA, this particular study was not hypothesis-driven. Follow-up research is planned to test the three-factor model identified here via factor analysis; this would meet another of Silvertown's guidelines (2009). The formal practice and empirical investigation of AAI is relatively new and there are many questions to be answered. This application of the citizen-science approach suggests practitioners are willing and excited to collaborate, and the data may be similar in quality to laboratory studies. Further testing of this method for AAI research is warranted.

References

Altman, D. G. (1991). Mathematics for kappa. In D. Altman (Ed.), *Practical statistics for medical research* (pp. 406–407). London: Chapman & Hall.

Barker, S. B., Knisely, J. S., McCain, N. L., & Best, A. M. (2005). Measuring stress and immune response in healthcare professionals following interaction with a therapy dog: A pilot study. *Psychological Reports, 96*(3), 713–729.

Bensky, M. K., Gosling, S. D., & Sinn, D. L. (2013). The world from a dog's point of view: A review and synthesis of dog cognition research. *Advanced Studies in Behavior, 45*, 209–406.

Bird, T. J., Bates, A. E., Lefcheck, J. S., Hill, N. A., Thomson, R. J., Edgar, G. J., et al. (2014). Statistical solutions for error and bias in global citizen science datasets. *Biological Conservation, 173*, 144–154.

Bonney, R., Ballard, H., Jordan, R., McCallie, E., Phillips, T., Shirk, J., & Wilderman, C.C. (2009). *Defining the field and assessing its potential for informal science education*. A CAISE Inquiry Group Report. Center for Advancement of Informal Science Education (CAISE), Washington, DC.

Brunner, J. (2004). Life as narrative. *Social Research, 71*, 691–711.

Burgess, H. K., DeBey, L. B., Froehlich, H. E., Schmidt, N., Theobald, E. J., Ettinger, A. K., et al. (2017). The science of citizen science: Exploring barriers to use as a primary research tool. *Biological Conservation, 208*, 113–120.

Chubak, J., & Hawkes, R. (2016). Animal-assisted activities: Results from a survey of top-ranked pediatric oncology hospitals. *Journal of Pediatric Oncology Nursing, 33*(4), 289–296.

Citizen-Science Association. (2019). *Home page*. www.citizen-science.org.

Coleman, J., Green, B., Garthe, R., Worthington, E., Barker, S., & Ingram, K. (2016). The Coleman dog attitude scale (C-DAS): Development, refinement, validation, and reliability. *Applied Animal Behaviour Science, 176*, 77–86.

Cooper, C. (2016). *Citizen science: How ordinary people are changing the face of discovery*. New York, NY: Overlook Press.

Equine-Assisted Growth and Learning Association. (2019). Our organization. Retrieved from https://www.eagala.org/org.

Fratkin, J., & Baker, S. C. (2013). The role of coat color and ear shape on the perception of personality in dogs. *Anthrozoös, 26*, 125–133.

Glenk, L. (2017). Current perspectives on therapy dog welfare in animal-assisted interventions. *Animals, 7*(2), 7.

Gray, P. B., & Young, S. M. (2011). Human–pet dynamics in cross-cultural perspective. *Anthrozoös, 24*(1), 17–30.

Haklay, M. (2013). Citizen science and volunteered geographic information: Overview and typology of participation. In *Crowdsourcing geographic knowledge* (pp. 105–122). Dordrecht: Springer.

Hecht, J., & Spicer Rice, E. (2015). Citizen science: A new direction in canine behavior research. *Behavioural Processes, 110*, 125–132.

Herzog, H. (2011). The impact of pets on human health and psychological well-being: Fact, fiction, or hypothesis? *Current Directions in Psychological Science, 20*(4), 236–239.

Krueger, K., Esch, L., & Byrne, R. (2019). Animal behaviour in a human world: A crowdsourcing study on horses that open door and gate mechanisms. *PLoS One, 14*(6), e0218954.

Ladd, D., & Barker, S. (2017). Dogs on call in a patient library. *Journal of Hospital Librarianship, 17*(1), 22–29.

Lavrakas, P. J. (2008). *Self-selection bias. Encyclopedia of survey research methods.* Thousand Oaks, CA: Sage.

Lynn, P. (2004). Sampling error. In *Encyclopedia of social science research methods.* Thousand Oaks, CA: Sage.

Mirkó, E., Kubinyi, E., Gácsi, M., & Miklósi, Á. (2012). Preliminary analysis of an adjective-based dog personality questionnaire developed to measure some aspects of personality in the domestic dog (Canis familiaris). *Applied Animal Behaviour Science, 138*(1–2), 88–98.

Pet Partners. (2019). *About.* Retrieved from https://petpartners.org/about-us/.

Porcher, J., Cousson-Gélie, F., & Dantzer, R. (2004). Affective components of the human-animal relationship in animal husbandry: Development and validation of a questionnaire. *Psychological Reports, 95*(1), 275–290.

Roetman, P., Tindle, H., & Litchfield, C. (2018). Management of pet cats: The impact of the cat tracker citizen science project in South Australia. *Animals, 8*(11), 190.

Shen, R. Z., Xiong, P., Chou, U. I., & Hall, B. J. (2018). "We need them as much as they need us": A systematic review of the qualitative evidence for possible mechanisms of effectiveness of animal-assisted intervention (AAI). *Complementary Therapies in Medicine, 41*, 203–207.

Shuller, D. Y., & McNamara, J. R. (1976). Expectancy factors in behavioral observation. *Behavior Therapy, 7*(4), 519–527.

Silvertown, J. (2009). A new dawn for citizen science. *Trends in Ecology & Evolution, 24*(9), 467–471.

Stewart, L., MacLean, E. L., Ivy, D., Woods, V., Cohen, E., Rodriguez, K., et al. (2015). Citizen science as a new tool in dog cognition research. *PLoS One, 10*(9), e0135176.

The Telegraph. (2013, February 20). "Houdini" horse escapes from stable and frees friends. Retrieved from https://www.youtube.com/watch?v=Aseg-w0hA_c&t=57s.

Thornton, G. C., & Zorich, S. (1980). Training to improve observer accuracy. *Journal of Applied Psychology, 65*(3), 351.

CHAPTER 7

Toward Empirical Thinking and Creative Inquiry

Abstract Here I summarize the main points covered in the book, discuss important limitations, and make suggestions for future research. Throughout this work, I have promoted inquiry into the process of animal-assisted intervention. Human–animal interaction (HAI) analysis was introduced as a potential practice to better understand interventions with animals and tie the animal to measured outcomes. Basic and applied studies provide examples of just how we can think empirically about the process of incorporating animals in interventions. After a brief summary of major points, this chapter discusses limitations of the research discussed and provides suggestions for improved investigation moving forward. Suggestions include operationalizing variables in a variety of ways, emphasizing sociocultural variables, considering animal autonomy and welfare, and reporting activities and findings responsibly.

Keywords Animal-assisted intervention • Human–animal interaction analysis

The purpose of this book has been to support researchers and practitioners in thinking empirically about animal-assisted intervention (AAI). After a brief overview of the history on AAI practice and research, specific methods and ideas were shared to inspire future work. If there is one theme that ties each topic together, it is the need for more analysis of the inner

A. K. Fournier, *Animal-Assisted Intervention*,
https://doi.org/10.1007/978-3-030-32972-3_7

workings of AAI. To that end, I've focused on studying the human–animal interaction (HAI) that occurs within AAI. This is important to understand the process, identify the animals' role in intervention, and support even more targeted, hypothesis-driven research. There is an underlying assumption in AAI that something is happening between the intervention animal and recipient and that the interaction or engagement causes or influences whatever outcome we measure. For example, if patients randomly assigned to receive canine-assisted occupational therapy end up with greater range of motion and improved functioning above and beyond that of a no-animal control condition, we assume the canine was a key ingredient in the intervention. We assume something happened between the humans and the canine(s) to cause the difference. But the truth is we wouldn't actually know why there was a difference between the intervention and control groups. We wouldn't know what the potent intervention components were and if the animal was one of them.

Intervention outcome is obviously an important area of study; research to date has focused on it almost exclusively. The evidence base is growing and indicates AAI can be an effective intervention for a range of purposes and populations. Over time, the scientific rigor of AAI outcome research has improved, moving from correlational to experimental methods. There have been a number of randomized controlled trials (RCTs), allowing for more definitive conclusions on the effects of AAI. On the whole, the outcome literature indicates positive effects and warrants continued research. The next phase of investigation must include a closer examination of the AAI process, with interactions between humans and animals as a key area of inquiry.

Each chapter in this book has covered a topic related to the AAI process. Chapter 2 introduced the concept of HAI analysis, introducing the Human–Animal Interaction Scale (HAIS) as a means for measuring behavioral interactions between humans and animals. This concept of examining behavioral HAI within AAI was then discussed throughout the book. Chapter 3 focused on HAI dose, providing examples of and making recommendations for studying the construct. To date, AAI dose has been rarely discussed, is limited to exchanges about session number and duration, and has not been tested for how it relates to intervention outcome. Research from our lab provides just a couple of examples of how dose could be operationalized and studied. Applying the medical model, dose–response curves were shown as a way to think about the relationship between HAI and outcome. The curves shared here suggest the relationship is curvilinear. Our research at the HAI laboratory indicates we cannot simply say "the more the merrier" when it comes to the effects of HAI quantity on psychological distress. Instead, our research suggests response increases with increasing dose to a certain point and then plateaus; there may be a point of diminishing returns.

The anodyne-agent model was introduced in Chaps. 4 and 5, providing a framework for thinking about two potential roles animals play in assisting intervention—eliciting an anodyne effect and serving as intervention agents. While not an explanatory theory, the model can be helpful in organizing research findings on the various interventions involving animals. Studies finding decreases in distress for students after an animal-related event on campus (e.g., Stewart et al. 2014), or increased happiness in nursing home residents who were visited by a therapy dog (e.g., Oliva et al. 2010) can be framed under the same umbrella of interaction with animals eliciting an anodyne effect, defined as decreased negative emotion (e.g., fear, anxiety, stress, loneliness) and/or increased positive emotion (e.g., happiness, calm, joy). Preliminary findings support this notion and warrant further investigation. Evidence of an anodyne effect was demonstrated in basic and applied studies, with both research participants and psychotherapy clients reporting improved mood as a function of interacting with animals. Combining related constructs under one superordinate construct can help streamline research, identifying one animal role versus several. This may be particularly useful in terms of animals as agents in the intervention process.

Note that practitioners and scholars do not use the term animal intervention, which might assume the animal *is* the intervention. Instead, we use the term animal-*assisted* intervention, suggesting there is an intervention aimed at one or more objectives and the animal assists in some way. Just as humans can serve as agents in behavior-change interventions (e.g., Fournier and Berry 2012; Geller et al. 1990; Ludwig and Geller 1999), animals can serve as agents in an intervention aimed at human health and well-being. The agent effect was supported with reports from AAI recipients and practitioners. Equine-assisted psychotherapy clients reported learning about their thoughts, feelings, and behaviors through interactions with horses. The animal served as the agent through which thought–feeling–behavior patterns were identified. This is an example of how a psychological intervention—cognitive-behavioral therapy—can be assisted by an animal. As mentioned earlier, the therapeutic goal and mechanism of change are similar for animal-assisted and office-based interventions. Incorporating animals is a modality or means through which an intervention can be delivered. Framing it this way, we could prevent the magical thinking or skepticism we sometimes see around AAI. There is a recognized intervention happening and an animal is being incorporated, rather than a vague notion that animals are good for us. Although scholarship suggests those of us in the field probably hold those assumptions (Herzog 2011), as professionals and scholars we need more objective language and more specific ideas about process and outcome. The anodyne-agent framework can be helpful in organizing the growing body of evidence on AAIs; a body of evidence that is currently quite broad.

Capturing a deeper understanding of AAI will require examination of many factors within the human recipient (e.g., personality, experience with and attitude toward animals, Geller 2016), intervention animal(s) (e.g., species, breed, temperament), animal handler/practitioner, and situation/setting. We will need creative measures for the large-scale data collection necessary to draw reliable conclusions about these factors. Citizen science was discussed in Chap. 6, as a means for large-scale AAI data collection. Data were gathered by Pet Partners practitioners. Their reports shed light on the range of interactions occurring between dogs and people in hospitals, nursing homes, and educational settings. Their perceptions of the animal's role in the intervention can be interpreted through the anodyne-agent model. Some practitioners saw their animal as providing an emotional benefit while others saw the animal as an aid in the actual intervention.

Confines and Future Considerations

Throughout the book, I've shared ideas and summarized studies on AAI. The research is described to provide ideas and inspire practitioners and researchers to think empirically about AAI. Thinking empirically means thinking critically, asking questions rather than relying on assumptions. With any empirical investigation, there are limitations to consider and those specific to each study have been mentioned within the chapters. In the spirit of thinking critically, there are also broader limitations to this research program as a whole that should be considered.

Scope

AAI is a broad field, with many questions to be answered through research. As is probably clear by now, my bias is to focus on the AAI process. I feel we need to understand how animals assist interventions, particularly if we want to make claims about the "healing power of animals" or the "power of pets" (Seppala 2017). In studying the process, I have focused on HAI, and defined HAI as the specific behaviors that occur between humans and animals during an intervention. However, there are other elements in the AAI process and other ways to define HAI.

Animals are incorporated into interventions for a variety of human benefits, including physical and mental health and functioning. As a psychologist, I tend to focus on psychology and psychotherapeutic mental-health interventions. Although I have referenced literature in the book from fields like occupational therapy and nursing, the empirical work shared throughout is centered on psychological intervention and outcome. Still, the ideas could be applied to and should be tested in other fields. For example, the examination of AAI dose through dose–response curves could be conducted within the physical-therapy field. Rather than response being based on a psychological outcome it could be based on physical functioning (e.g., the percentage of patients with improved range of motion per dose).

Moving forward as a field, we need both breadth and depth. There is room for inquiry into AAI process and outcome, with a range of interventions and populations. We need answers to a wide range of questions. Individual studies, however, should target more narrow, specific research questions. Outcome measures should connect to the objectives of the intervention. If a dog is incorporated into psychotherapy addressing depression, the outcome to measure is mood and other symptoms of depression. If an animal visiting is meant to distract a hospital patient from the distress of their treatment, the variable to measure is attention, distraction, or focus. Then research is needed to understand which role the animal played in that outcome. My bias is that an analysis of the interactions occurring between the client/patient and the intervention animal is important in identifying the animal's role.

HAI Analysis

Throughout the book, I have discussed the importance of analyzing the interactions that occur in AAI, and the data I've shared were gathered via the HAIS. Thinking critically about the instrument, there are some areas where it falls short, leaving the door open for other measures that exist or are awaiting development. While the HAI analysis reviewed here may encourage practitioners and researchers to think empirically about AAI, it is just one way of looking at the interactions that occur between humans and animals. The HAIS provides a means for recording behavioral HAI; it does not allow for gathering information on other aspects of interaction (e.g., emotional engagement). And while the measure includes a variety of behaviors that can be emitted by humans and animals during interaction, many of the behaviors could be further specified. For example, there are various ways to *pet* an animal. *Talking* to an animal can look quite different depending on rate, tone, and content of speech. So, analysis of behavioral HAI may need to be more nuanced than the HAIS allows.

The HAIS requires a certain level of recall to record behaviors that occurred in a period of interaction once the episode is over. To that end, we must ask whether people remember what happened during a session accurately. With the Pet Partners study discussed in Chap. 6, some session logs were completed several days later. Even when completed immediately, processes occurring during an AAI could make it difficult to notice and remember specific behaviors. On a related note, the rating system may be an opportunity for error. My rating an interaction as a 2 may be your 3. In the laboratory we notice ratings are consistently higher for the client experiencing the HAI than for researchers observing the HAI. While the client's subjective perception is important, some studies may require a more objective measure. In those cases, an observation coding tool, such as the Observation of Human–Animal Interaction for Research (OHAIRE) coding tool (Guérin et al. 2018; O'Haire et al. 2013) could be useful.

Anything we do before, during, or after an intervention can potentially impact the intervention process and outcome. In psychotherapy, it was once believed that practitioners should be a "blank slate" so as not to allow the therapist to influence the client's experience (Brill 1921). Regarding HAI analysis, asking people to report on specific behaviors—whether clients or practitioners—could make those behaviors seem normal or expected. These expectations could then shape behavior in future sessions. This arrives at the delicate balance between respecting and trusting the intervention process and examining the process to further science. Eagala suggests that effects of an equine-assisted psychotherapy session can occur after "soak time," or a period of time in which the client can reflect on happenings in the session (Eagala 2019). When asked about significant moments in psychotherapy, clients report that processing between sessions is an important part of their therapeutic process (Levitt et al. 2006).

In this context, we can imagine that asking clients to complete any self-report measure after a session could impact the way they reflect on and process session content. With regard to HAI analysis, completing the HAIS could interrupt the natural process following a session, prompting additional or alternative thoughts or feelings. For example, perhaps an animal-assisted psychotherapy session addressing grief left a client thinking about the life cycle of all animals, but completing the HAIS shifted their focus to specific behaviors that occurred in the session and their meaning. Personally, I struggle with this as a scientist-practitioner. Understanding a process can require breaking it down and studying the intricate details in a systematic fashion. But in doing so, we might interrupt the natural process, which impacts the intervention and the data gathered on that intervention. Fleet et al. (2016) discuss the conflict between a reductionist, nomothetic approach to understanding human behavior and a genuine understanding of the therapeutic process. I am fortunate to have practitioner colleagues who share their experiences and allow for archival research to identify patterns and develop research questions that can then be tested in the laboratory with nonclinical samples. Experimental findings are then shared with the practitioners for interpretation through both scientist and practitioner lenses. Over time, this has helped me develop programmatic, rather than serendipitous, research. For the practitioners, it has facilitated empirical thinking about their AAI practice, helping them gather data and learn more about their clients, therapy animals, and practice.

Sociocultural Variables and Social Justice Issues

The research examples provided here are limited in diversity, all conducted from one corner of the world. We know that human–animal relationships differ across cultures. Our attitudes and beliefs about animals are shaped by our cultural background (Harris 1974). Animal roles are socially constructed (Foucault 1970; Noske 1989); we see them based on human definitions and these definitions differ across cultures. Dogs are constructed as food in some parts of the world and as family members in others. Working in a pasture with horses may result in a different outcome based on one's knowledge of or experience with horses. Thinking empirically about AAI must include an appreciation for and examination of social and cultural variables. These can include the impact of social identity on AAI process and outcome. For example, are interventions with animals applied or experienced differently based on the client's gender, race, orientation, or social class? Anecdotally, my colleagues and I have observed differences. Some participants in equine-assisted psychotherapy respond quite strongly to wildlife entering the session space (e.g., an eagle flying over or a fox walking through the pasture), giving it special meaning and shifting the course of the session. Others may notice it, attribute no particular meaning, and continue with the session as they were. These differences in attention and meaning could be culturally based. Anecdotally, international students in our laboratory have reported less experience with pet dogs or cats than their American counterparts. As a result, these students might interact less with the animals. The specific interactive behaviors could differ as well. HAI may be more casual for someone with less experience (e.g., *watching* the animal) and more active or affectionate for someone with more experience (e.g., *playing with*, *hugging*, or *kissing* the animal). In addition, the impact of certain interactions could be different for someone with less animal experience; the effect of an animal initiating interaction could increase anxiety rather than decrease it. These are important issues to study empirically. Citizen science can be helpful in casting a wide net, gathering data on interactions between humans and animals all over the world. In addition to practitioners gathering data on AAI, pet owners could provide data on interactions between themselves and their pet.

Regarding demographics of the studies described here, our samples were largely women, consistent with women's positive attitudes toward animals (Herzog 2007), research on AAI (Berget and Grepperud 2011), and anthrozoology in general (e.g., DeMello 2012). Samples were also mostly White. Data on pet-keeping in general indicate racial disparities, with Whites making up the majority of the pet-keeping population in some surveys. Surveys on pet ownership in the U.S. have found the ratio of pet ownership in White versus Black respondents to be 64% versus 30% (Pew Research Center 2006) and 75% vs. 37% (Melson 2001).

Risley-Curtiss and colleagues (2006) surveyed American households on pet ownership, examining the human–animal bond in the context of ethnic diversity. Their results suggested different rates of pet-keeping among racial/ethnic groups. The survey found that Native American respondents had the highest rates of pet ownership at 73.5%, followed by Whites (65.0%), people of Hispanic/Spanish heritage (56.9%), people who identified as African American or Black (40.9%), Pacific Islanders (40%), and Asian people (37.5%). There were some differences regarding which animals people kept as pets. Native American respondents were more likely than other groups to report having fish as pets, and Hispanic respondents were less likely than other groups to have cats. There were also some important similarities. For all groups, dogs were the most common pet. When asked about their relationship with their pet(s) and what it offered them, there were no differences in the perception that pets offered emotional support, companionship, and unconditional love. There were also no differences in the perception of pets as members of the family. While pet ownership is not the same as being an AAI research practitioner (e.g., Pet Partner study), a research participant (e.g., university laboratory study), or an AAI recipient (e.g., AAI client), we can glean some sense of the variability in HAI experiences from these studies on pet-keeping. The data suggest that people from different backgrounds have differing levels of experience with animals; those experiences could impact the process or outcome of an AAI.

Beyond different experiences with animals in general, AAI could resonate quite differently for one group versus another, based on histories of power and oppression around people, nature, and animals. Jones and Segal (2018) discuss ecopsychology's intersection with settler colonialism. Ecopsychology practice or ecotherapy involves nature connection practices focused on cultivating relationships with the "more-than-human world" (i.e., animals and nature) (Abram 1996; Cohen 1997). Ecopsychology practices include therapies or activities wherein the crux of an intervention is connection with nature, involving direct contact with the natural world and occurring outside on the land. It includes animal-assisted therapy (AAT) among other practices (e.g., horticulture therapy, wilderness therapy, forest bathing). Settler colonialism is "a form of colonization in which outsiders come to land inhabited by Indigenous peoples and claim it as their own new home" (Tuck et al. 2014, p. 8). Scholars suggest programs aimed at reconnecting people with the land and natural world reproduce the myths of settler innocence and peacemaker, and ignore the displacement of Indigenous peoples from the settings in which ecopsychology practices occur (Jones and Segal 2018; McLean 2013). Essentially, a case is made that non-Indigenous, White settler practitioners employing nature (e.g., land, plants, animals, earth) in treatment is an act of present-day colonialism.

Taken together, we can imagine that people will experience interactions with animals differently based on personal factors, including social and cultural identities. Our work should include strategic methods to recruit diverse participant pools, investigate the relationships between sociocultural variables and HAI/AAI, and account for the field's broad implications in the context of historical and current arrangements of people, animals, and nature.

Animal Autonomy and Welfare

The focus of this book has been on the humans involved in AAI. This is consistent with the bulk of the research to date; studies focus on the experience and outcome for human intervention recipients. The studies I've described throughout the book also focused heavily on the human experience. Dose was discussed as it relates to human outcomes; the anodyne-agent model is a framework for understanding animal roles in impacting subjective distress and therapeutic process from the human client/patient perspective. But what about the animals?

Recently, there has been an increased focus on the welfare of therapy animals. Scholars have expressed a concern for the health and well-being of animals used in interventions (Serpell et al. 2010). Concerns include loss of freedom and choice, stress, and fatigue. Glenk (2017) conducted a literature review on therapy dog welfare in AAI. Although variability across AAI programs precluded declaration of any reliable effects, studies showed evidence of negative effects for the therapy dogs. Specifically, dogs demonstrated changes in salivary cortisol, stereotypic autogrooming, and stress-related behaviors; this was particularly true if the intervention recipients were children under age 12.

Although practitioners and researchers are beginning to consider more closely intervention animals' well-being, we are still in need of standardization and guidelines. We do not have research-based recommendations for the appropriate frequency and duration of sessions, particularly for animals of a specific species, condition, or age (Enders-Slegers et al. 2019). It seems to me the need for more research on intervention animal welfare could be carried out in two ways: (1) research on intervention animal welfare is conducted for the sake of it, and (2) research targeting *human* process and/or outcome should also always include measuring variables related to the *animal* process and/or outcome. Adding an element of the animal perspective to the plethora of research already happening on the human perspective would quickly increase the research base on intervention animal welfare. Again, my bias is that we need to understand how the AAI process impacts the animal's welfare just as much as the welfare outcome itself. To best avoid harm to animals employed in interventions, we need to understand not just *if* the process impacts them, but *how*.

Responsible Reporting

Despite the promising findings of AAI outcome research, we cannot assume that AAI is always effective. Even treatments with a strong evidence base can have poor results from time to time. And although I have focused on my own research and reviewed previous studies with promising findings, that is not always the case. Chapter 4 briefly discussed this issue, mentioning several studies in which an anodyne effect was the goal but results showed no difference in comparison to other nonanimal interventions. There are likely many more studies with poor results that never get published, something we refer to as the file-drawer problem (Rosenthal 1979). Herzog (2014) discusses this issue, pointing out the discrepancy between studies showing positive results and the actual meaning of small effect sizes in AAI research. It is incumbent upon us as practitioners and researchers to examine our practices critically and to report on intervention processes and outcomes honestly. A thorough account includes a discussion of adverse effects and insignificant findings.

Conclusion

When it comes to thinking empirically about AAI, the world is our oyster. We have many questions to ponder and innumerable routes of investigation. My hope is that this book has provided ideas for critical thinking and creative inquiry into the ways humans and animals engage for health and well-being. I encourage you to employ your curiosity and share all that you learn. Together, we can develop a clearer understanding of interventions involving animals.

References

Abram, D. (1996). *Spell of the sensuous.* New York, NY: Vintage Books.

Berget, B., & Grepperud, S. (2011). Animal-assisted interventions for psychiatric patients: Beliefs in treatment effects among practitioners. *European Journal of Integrative Medicine, 3*(2), e91–e96.

Brill, A. A. (1921). *Basic principles of psychoanalysis.* New York, NY: University Press of America.

Cohen, M. (1997). *Reconnecting with nature: Finding wellness through rebuilding your bond with earth* (2nd ed.). Friday Harbour, WA: Ecopress.

DeMello, M. (2012). *Animals and society: An introduction to human-animal studies.* New York, NY: Columbia University Press.

Enders-Slegers, M. J., Hediger, K., Beetz, A., Jegatheesan, B., & Turner, D. (2019). Animal-assisted intervention within an international perspective: Trends, research, and practices. In A. H. Fine (Ed.), *Handbook on animal-assisted therapy: Foundations and guidelines for animal-assisted interventions* (5th ed., pp. 465–478). San Diego, CA: Elsevier.

Equine-Assisted Growth and Learning Association. (2019). *Fundamentals of the Eagala model: Becoming an Eagala certified professional.* Santaquin, UT: Eagala.

Fleet, D., Burton, A., Reeves, A., & DasGupta, M. P. (2016). A case for taking the dual role of counselor-researcher in qualitative research. *Qualitative Research in Psychology, 13*(4), 328–346.

Foucault, M. (1970). *The order of things: An archaeology of the human sciences.* New York: Pantheon.

Fournier, A. K., & Berry, T. D. (2012). Effects of response cost and socially-assisted interventions on hand hygiene behavior of university students. *Behavior and Social Issues, 21*, 152–164. https://doi.org/10.5210/bsi.v.21i0.3979.

Geller, K. S. (2016). The AC4P power of pets. In E. S. Geller (Ed.), *Applied psychology: Actively caring for people* (pp. 623–644). New York, NY: Cambridge University Press.

Geller, E. S., Berry, T. D., Ludwig, T. D., Evans, R. E., Gilmore, M. R., & Clarke, S. W. (1990). A conceptual framework for developing and evaluating behavior change interventions for injury control. *Health Education Research, 5*(2), 125–137.

Glenk, L. (2017). Current perspectives on therapy dog welfare in animal-assisted interventions. *Animals, 7*(2), 7.

Guérin, N. A., Gabriels, R. L., Germone, M. M., Schuck, S. E., Traynor, A., Thomas, K. M., et al. (2018). Reliability and validity assessment of the observation of human-animal interaction for research (OHAIRE) behavior coding tool. *Frontiers in Veterinary Science, 5.*

Harris, M. (1974). *Cows, pigs, wars, and witches: The riddles of culture.* New York, NY: Vintage Books.

Herzog, H. (2007). Gender differences in human-animal interactions: A review. *Anthrozoös, 20*(1), 7–21.

Herzog, H. (2011). The impact of pets on human health and psychological well-being: Fact, fiction, or hypothesis? *Current Directions in Psychological Science, 20*(4), 236–239.

Herzog, H. (2014, November 17). Does animal-assisted therapy really work? What clinical trials reveal about the effectiveness of four-legged therapists. *Psychology Today.* Retrieved from https://www.psychology today.com/us/blog/animals-and-us/201411/does-animal-assisted-therapy-really-work.

Jones, A. T., & Segal, D. S. (2018). Unsettling ecopsychology: Addressing settler colonialism in ecopsychology practice. *Ecopsychology, 10*(3), 127–136.

Levitt, H., Butler, M., & Hill, T. (2006). What clients find helpful in psychotherapy: Developing principles for facilitating moment-to-moment change. *Journal of Counseling Psychology, 53*(3), 314.

Ludwig, T. D., & Geller, E. S. (1999). Behavior change among agents of a community safety program: Pizza deliverers advocate community safety belt use. *Journal of Organizational Behavior Management, 19*(2), 3–24.

McLean, S. (2013). The whiteness of green: Racialization and environmental education. *Canadian Geographer, 57*, 354–362.

Melson, G. F. (2001). *Why the wild things are: Animals in the lives of children*. Cambridge, MA: Harvard University Press.

Noske, B. (1989). *Humans and other animals: Beyond the boundaries of anthropology*. London: Pluto.

O'Haire, M. E., McKenzie, S. J., Beck, A. M., & Slaughter, V. (2013). Social behaviors increase in children with autism in the presence of animals compared to toys. *PLoS One, 8*(2), e57010. https://doi.org/10.1371/journal.pone.0057010.

Oliva, V. N. L. S., Albuquerque, V. B., Silva, E. Y. T., Yamamoto, K. C. M., Costa, K. N., Silva, M. L. M., et al. (2010). Institutionalized elderly and animal assisted activities (AAA). *Revista Ciência em Extensão, 6*(2), 15–31.

Pew Research Center. (2006). *Gauging family intimacy: Dogs edge cats (dads trail both)*. A Social Trends Report. Washington, DC: Pew Research Center.

Risley-Curtiss, C., Holley, L. C., & Wolf, S. (2006). The animal-human bond and ethnic diversity. *Social Work, 51*(3), 257–268.

Rosenthal, R. (1979). The file drawer problem and tolerance for null results. *Psychological Bulletin, 86*(3), 638.

Seppala, E. (2017, July 11). How animals heal us and teach us: On the healing power of pets. *Psychology Today*. Retrieved from https://www.psychologytoday.com/us/blog/feeling-it/201707/how-animals-heal-us-and-teach-us.

Serpell, J. A., Coppinger, R., Fine, A. H., & Peralta, J. M. (2010). Welfare considerations in therapy and assistance animals. In A. H. Fine (Ed.), *Handbook on animal-assisted therapy* (pp. 481–503). Academic Press.

Stewart, L. A., Dispenza, F., Parker, L., Chang, C. Y., & Cunnien, T. (2014). A pilot study assessing the effectiveness of an animal-assisted outreach program. *Journal of Creativity in Mental Health, 9*(3), 332–345.

Tuck, E., McKenzie, M., & McCoy, K. (2014). Land education: Indigenous, postcolonial, and decolonizing perspectives on place and environmental education research. *Environmental Education Research, 20*(1), 1–23.

Appendix A: Human-Animal Interaction Scale—Participant Form[1]

[1] Scoring Instructions: Add items 1–12, then subtract items 13–14 for the Human Total. Sum items 15–20, then subtract items 21–24 for the Animal Total. Sum Human and Animal totals for the TOTAL HAI score.

A. K. Fournier, *Animal-Assisted Intervention*,
https://doi.org/10.1007/978-3-030-32972-3

Human-Animal Interaction Scale (HAIS)

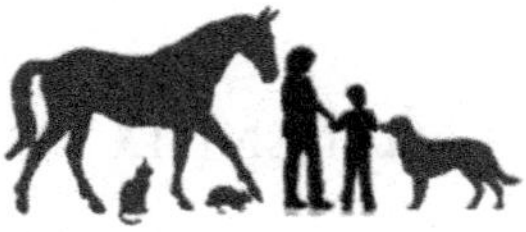

Name: ______________________________ Date: __________

Which animal(s) did you interact with? ________________________________

Instructions: For each **type** of interaction on the left, rate the **amount** of interaction you experienced on the right.

During the session, how much did YOU...	Not At All		A Moderate Amount		A Great Deal
1. Watch the animal(s)	0	1	2	3	4
2. Spend time near the animal(s)	0	1	2	3	4
3. Pet the animal(s)	0	1	2	3	4
4. Talk to the animal(s)	0	1	2	3	4
5. Hug the animal(s)	0	1	2	3	4
6. Play with the animal(s)	0	1	2	3	4
7. Kiss the animal(s)	0	1	2	3	4
8. Groom the animal(s)	0	1	2	3	4
9. Offer food to the animal(s)	0	1	2	3	4
10. Attempt Tricks or Training with the animal(s)	0	1	2	3	4
11. Hold the animal(s)	0	1	2	3	4
12. Take Pictures of or with the animal(s)	0	1	2	3	4
13. Decline or avoid interaction with the animal(s)	0	1	2	3	4
14. Behave aggressively toward the animal(s)	0	1	2	3	4
Human Total					
During the session, how much did THE ANIMAL(S)...	Not At All		Moderate Amount		A Great Deal
15. Initiate friendly interaction with you	0	1	2	3	4
16. Make friendly sounds	0	1	2	3	4
17. Accept food from you	0	1	2	3	4
18. Obey tricks or training	0	1	2	3	4
19. Sniff or smell you	0	1	2	3	4
20. Lick you	0	1	2	3	4
21. Make unfriendly sounds	0	1	2	3	4
22. Behave aggressively toward you	0	1	2	3	4
23. Cause a mess or inconvenience for you	0	1	2	3	4
24. Decline or avoid interaction with you	0	1	2	3	4
Animal Total					
TOTAL					

25. Did you enjoy interacting with the animal(s) today?	0	1	2	3	4
26. Did you make an emotional connection with the animal(s)?	0	1	2	3	4

Appendix B: Human-Animal Interaction Scale—Observer Form

Human-Animal Interaction Scale (HAIS) - Observer Form

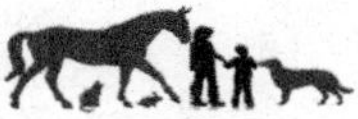

Rater:	Animal:	Rating	Notes
Instructions: After observing an episode or session of human-animal interaction, rate each behavior according to the % of the episode in which the behavior was observed.			
Item	**Operational Definition**		
How much did the client/participant…		**0-4**	
1. Watch the animal(s)	Eyes directed toward the animal		
2. Spend time near the animal(s)	Within arm's reach		
3. Pet the animal(s)	Hand on animal, moves from one point to another (pat or pet)		
4. Talk to the animal(s)	non-command Verbal behavior toward the animal		
5. Play with the animal(s)	Attempts to play		
6. Hug the animal(s)	Brings the animal close to their heart in an embrace		
7. Kiss the animal(s)	Lips on animal, puckered		
8. Groom the animal(s)	Brushing, combing, washing, clipping		
9. Offer food to the animal(s)	Holds or places food in front of the animal		
10. Attempt tricks or training with the animal(s)	Attempts tricks/obedience, verbal and physical commands		
11. Hold the animal(s)	Animal is physically on the person's body		
12. Take pictures of or with the animal(s)	Takes pictures or video with phone or camera		
13. Decline or avoid interaction w the animal(s)ith	Moves away from or pushes animal away		
14. Behave aggressively toward the animal(s)	Verbally Aggressive or physically aggressive (yell, hit, intimidate)		
How much did the animal…		**0-4**	
15. Initiate friendly interaction with the client/participant	Approach, touch, gesture,		
16. Make friendly sounds	Pant, purr, bark, friendly whine		
17. Accept food from the client/participant	Eats food participant puts in front of them		
18. Obey tricks or training with the client/participant	Obeys command given, verbal or physical		
19. Sniff or smell the client/participant	Sniffs or smells on or in direction of participant		
20. Lick the client/participant	Tongue on person in friendly way		
21. Make unfriendly sounds	Bark, growl, screach, howl		
22. Behave aggressively toward the client/participant	Bite, claw, jump on, lunge at		
23. Make a mess or inconvenience for the client/participant	Urinate, defecate, knock things over, spill, chewing objects		
24. Decline or Avoid interaction with the client/participant	Moves away from, hides		

Ratings for % of the time

0 = did not occur 1 = up to 25% 2 = 25-50% 3 = 50-75% 4 = >75%

A. K. Fournier, *Animal-Assisted Intervention*,
https://doi.org/10.1007/978-3-030-32972-3

Index[1]

[1] Note: Page numbers followed by 'n' refer to notes.

A. K. Fournier, *Animal-Assisted Intervention*,
https://doi.org/10.1007/978-3-030-32972-3

Made in the USA
Monee, IL
05 November 2026

67811182R00095